"M.O.P. was literally life saving for my

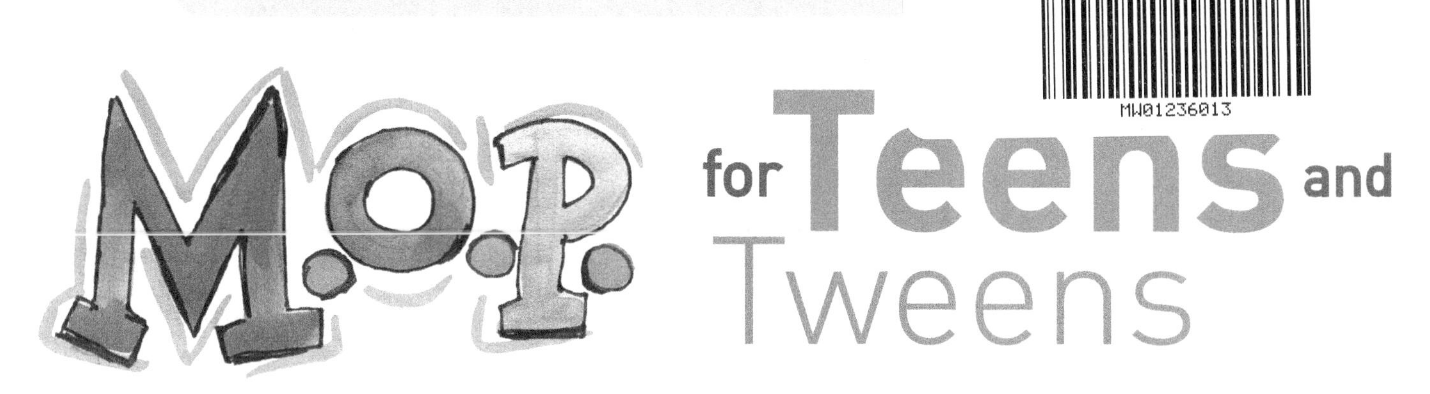

M.O.P. for Teens and Tweens

The Science-Based Way to STOP Bedwetting and Encopresis for Ages 10 to 18

Reviewed and Approved by Teens!

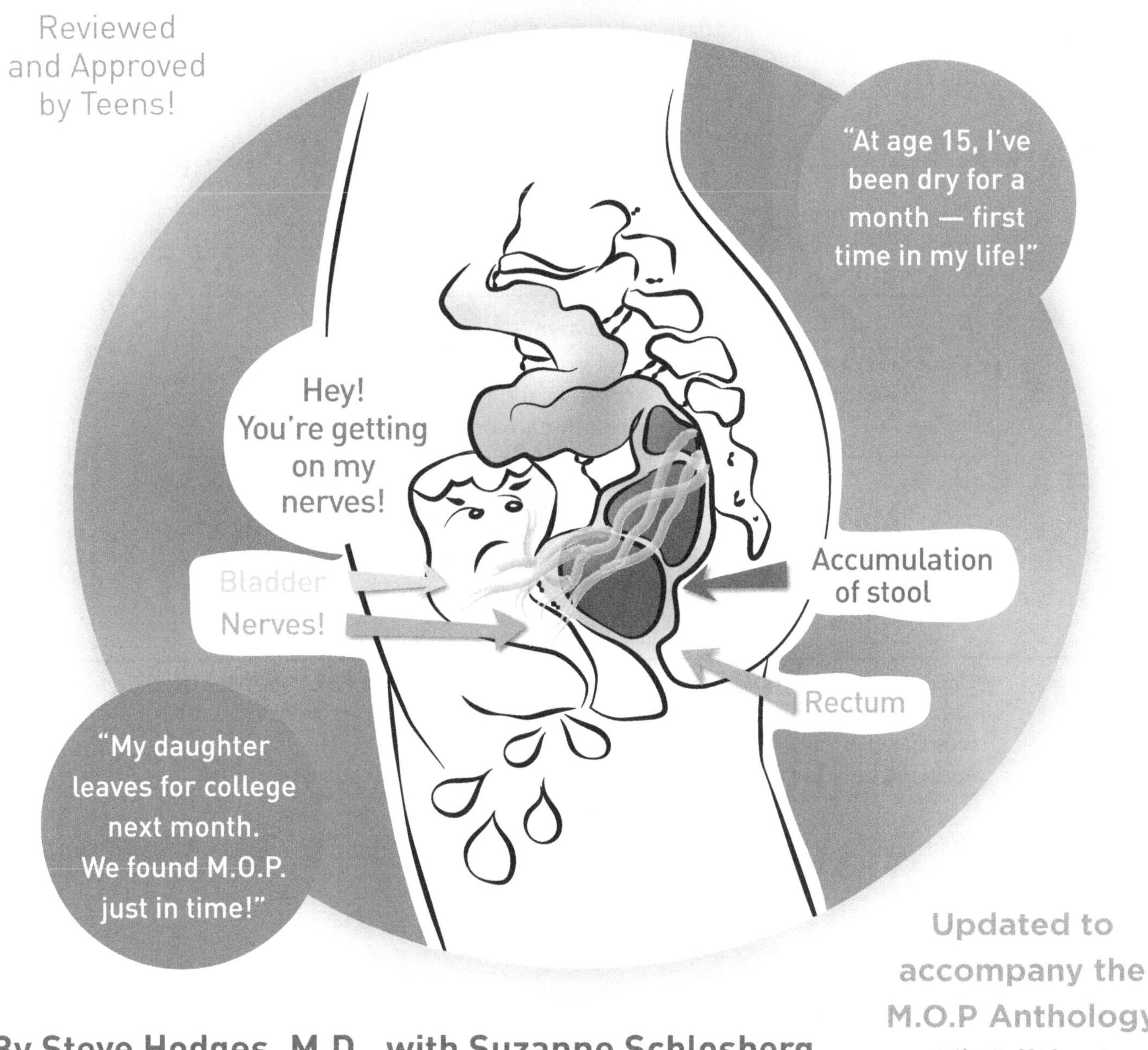

Updated to accompany the M.O.P Anthology 5th Edition!

By Steve Hodges, M.D., with Suzanne Schlosberg

Illustrations by Cristina Acosta and Mark Beech

Also written by Steve Hodges, M.D., and Suzanne Schlosberg

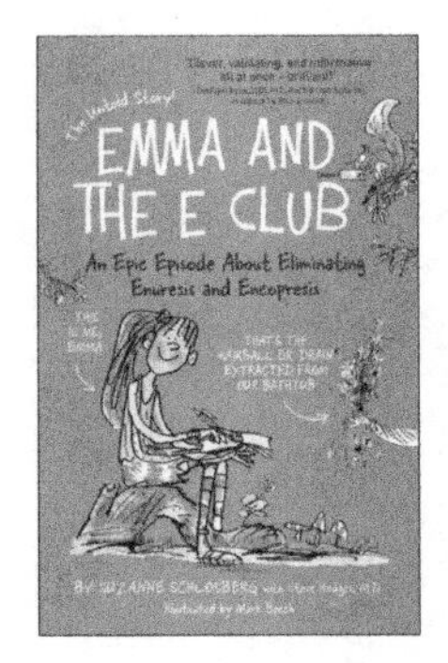

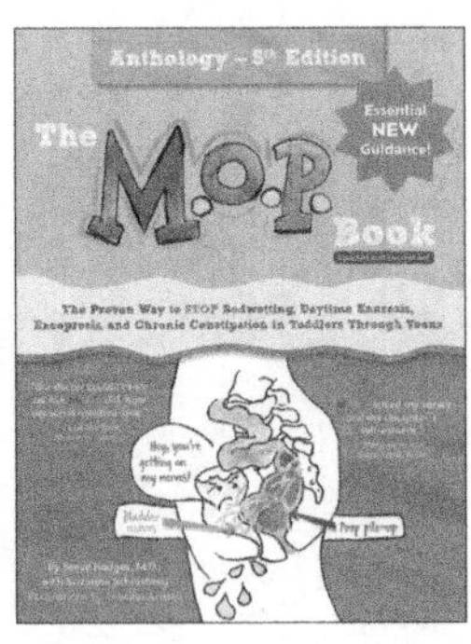

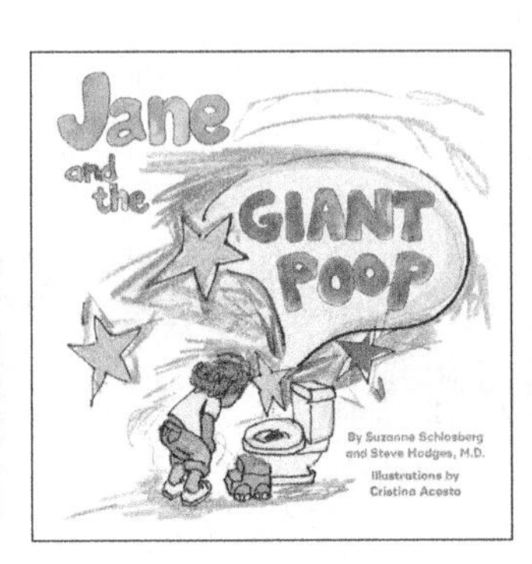

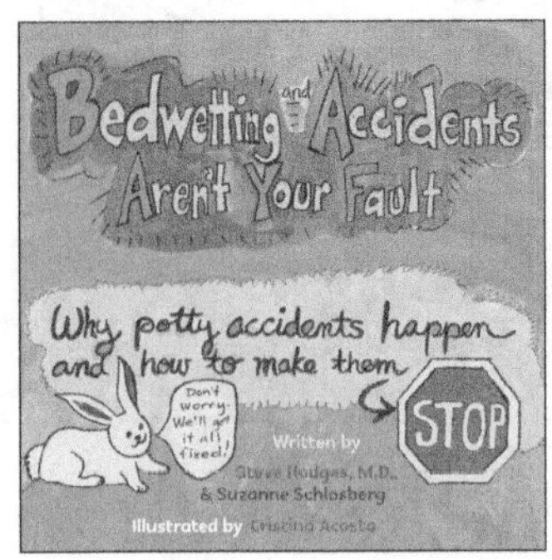

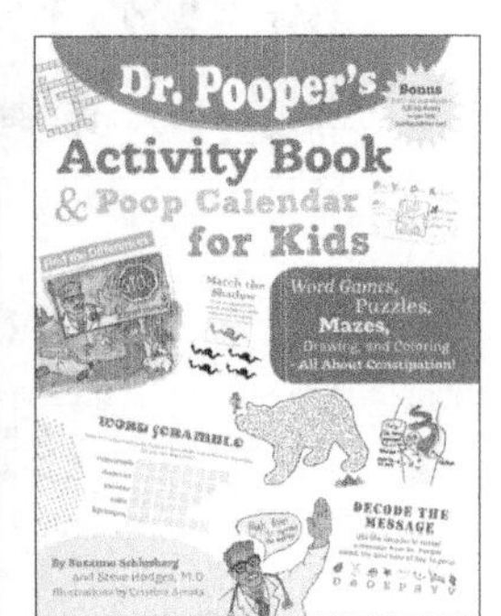

Available in paperback on amazon or for instant download at

BedwettingAndAccidents.com

Disclaimer

The information contained in this book is intended to supplement, not substitute for, the expertise and judgment of your physician or other health-care professional.

M.O.P. for Teens and Tweens

Book design: DyanRothDesign.com

O'Regan Press

Library of Congress Cataloging-in-Publication Data is available on file.

979-8-9866795-4-9

Important Note!

This short guide is not a substitute for *The M.O.P. Anthology 5th Edition*.

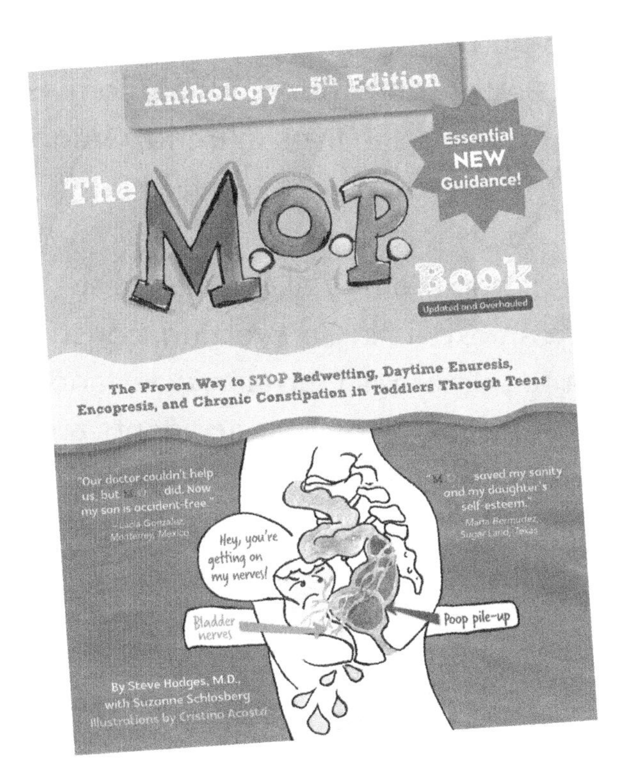

The *Anthology* explains the five M.O.P. variations in detail and provides essential guidance on choosing, using, and dosing enemas and laxatives. Do not implement M.O.P. without the *Anthology 5th Edition*!

M.O.P. for Teens and Tweens is an overview of M.O.P. written for middle school and high-school students.

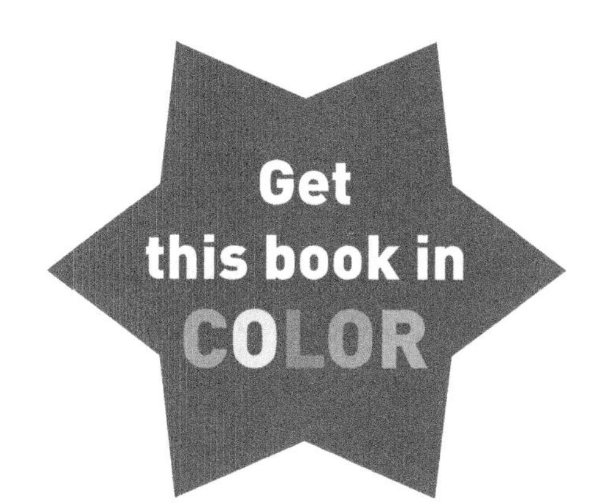

If you would like a free PDF in color, email your amazon receipt or a photo of the book to suzanne@bedwettingandaccidents.com.

About the Authors

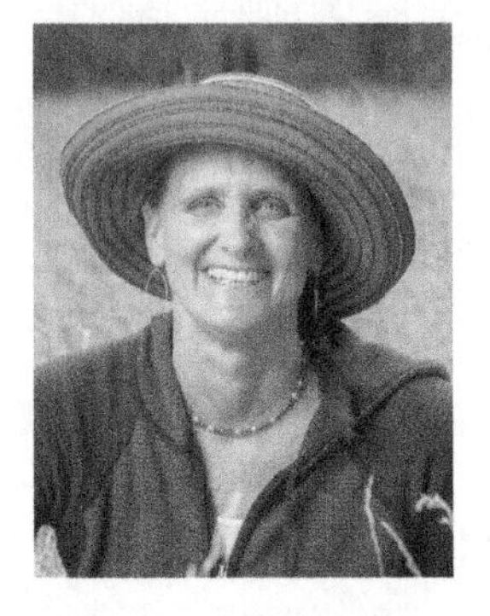

Suzanne Schlosberg

Suzanne is a health and parenting writer who specializes in translating medical mumbo jumbo into stuff that's fun to read. Years ago, she potty-trained her twin boys too early and used Steve Hodges' methods to undo the damage. Author or co-author of 20 books and countless articles, Suzanne is co-founder of BedwettingAndAccidents.com. Her website is SuzanneSchlosbergWrites.com. She lives in Bend, Oregon.

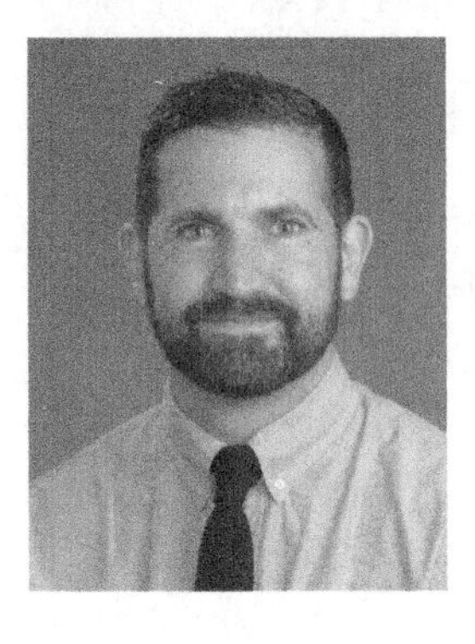

Steve Hodges, M.D.

Steve Hodges is a professor of pediatric urology at Wake Forest University School of Medicine and an expert in bedwetting, constipation, and potty training. He has authored numerous journal articles and co-authored six books. His mission is to assure kids that accidents are never their fault. A dad of three, he lives in Winston-Salem, North Carolina and blogs at BedwettingAndAccidents.com.

About the Artists

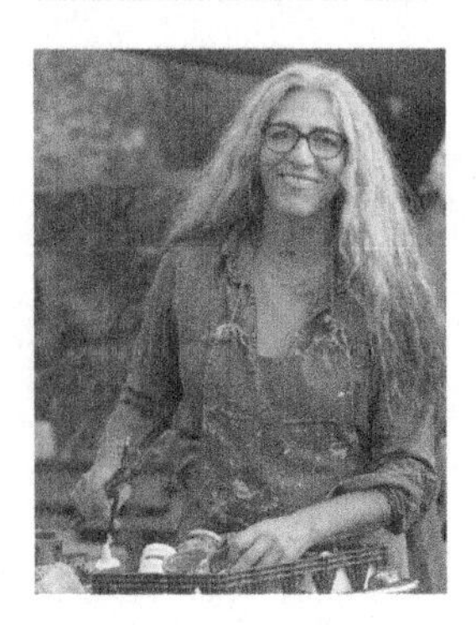

Cristina Acosta

Cristina is a painter, designer, and architectural color expert known for her bold use of color. Cristina has taught painting and drawing and exhibited in galleries throughout the West. On the side, she illustrates the content for BedwettingAndAccidents.com. Her clever take on childhood constipation brings much-needed humor and compassion to the subject. Cristina lives in La Quinta, California. Her website is CristinaAcosta.com.

Mark Beech

Mark Beech is a U.K.-based illustrator whose work is popular in the world of children's publishing. Mark has been illustrating professionally for over 20 years and has been scribbling since he was old enough to hold a pen. He has illustrated books for Sir Terry Pratchett, Jo Nesbo, Anthony Horowitz, and Enid Blyton, to name a few. *Emma and the E Club* was Mark's first foray into the world of constipation. You can see more of Mark's work at MarkBeechIllustration.com.

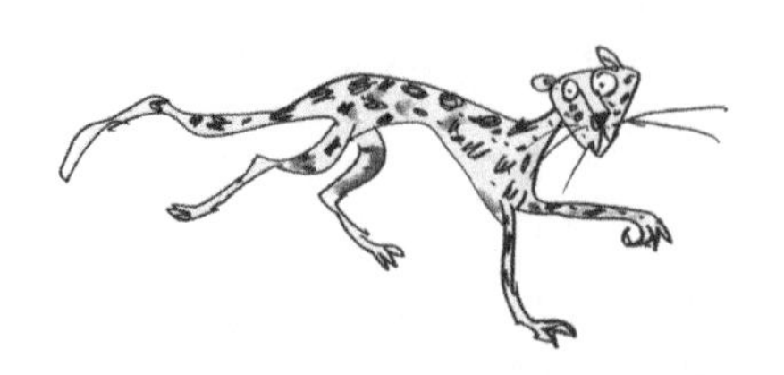

TABLE OF CONTENTS

INTRODUCTION

Yes, We Can Fix This!

My favorite patients are the teenagers. When I look ahead to the next day's schedule, I glance at the birthdates of my upcoming patients. Chances are, I'll have at least a couple of middle-school or high-school students on the list. I look forward to seeing these kids because I know I can brighten their day — not with false hope but with a triple dose of science-based reality: *Your condition is common. It's not your fault. It's totally fixable.*

Teens with bedwetting and/or daytime accidents have been dealt a crummy hand. They have a treatable condition that hasn't been treated properly. Some of my patients were never treated at all; they were simply assured, year after year, by doctor after doctor, "Don't worry, it's normal, you'll outgrow it."

Many have endured years of useless remedies — alarms, bladder medications, liquid restrictions, hypnosis, gluten-free diets, dairy-free diets, sugar-free diets, chiropractic, midnight wake-ups, bribery, rewards, counseling for stress and anxiety. I've even had patients who were sprayed with water in the middle of the night as part of a very misguided treatment.

I'm sure I don't need to tell you that middle-school and high-school students with bedwetting live in a state of distress — avoiding sleepovers, worried that friends will learn their secret, terrified the accidents won't stop before college. I run a private Facebook support group for parents of teens and tweens with these conditions, and when I created an anonymous survey, I heard plenty about how lousy their kids feel. For example:

> *"Our son feels like something is wrong with him, and this will never end."*
>
> *"Our son feels embarrassed, He's had accidents at school and pretends he spilled something on his pants."*

One mom said her daughter was teased after wetting her pants at church camp. Another reported her son feels sad every time he says no to a sleepover or sports camp, knowing his friends can go on overnights without a worry. "He thinks it's his fault, even though we've always told him it's not."

For years, these kids have shouldered shame and blame for a condition beyond their control, and have heard many groundless statements from doctors:

"You're a deep sleeper, but don't worry — no one goes to college wetting the bed."

"You have a small bladder. Just pee every 2 hours."

"You must like greasy foods. You need to eat healthier."

"Your bladder is underdeveloped."

"Your bladder muscles are overdeveloped."

"You're allergic to wheat."

"Try nightly affirmations and a bedwetting alarm."

"You probably have a hormone imbalance."

"It's probably stress — see a therapist."

If you're a teen or tween with enuresis (daytime or nighttime wetting) and/or encopresis (poop accidents), I'll bet you've heard these lines before. Here's what you should have been told instead: Enuresis and encopresis are caused by chronic constipation. What exactly does that mean? Well, constipation has a lot of definitions, many of them incorrect. What I'm talking about is a pile-up of stool — aka poop — in your rectum, which is the last section of your colon, located just before your anus (butthole!).

"When my mom first suggested I use enemas, I was terrified. But I soon realized enemas aren't scary at all. I've wet the bed my whole life. Now, at 15, I'm finally dry!"

Here's how I explain things to my patients: When you poop, your rectum is not completely emptying. Some stool ends up in the toilet, but some remains in your rectum. Gradually, the remaining stool piles up. This accumulation stretches your rectum — a lot. In fact, your rectum might be twice as wide as usual. Or wider! When your rectum is enlarged like this, it presses against your bladder. In otherwise healthy kids, a stretched rectum is responsible for about 99% of bedwetting cases and daytime pee accidents and 100% of encopresis cases. Yet in so many cases, nobody realizes the kid's rectum is clogged!

In this guide, I will explain exactly how constipation triggers accidents, why you haven't heard this explanation before, and how an X-Ray can prove whether or not your rectum has been stretched. But for the moment, trust me: That's what's going on.

TIP FROM A TEEN:

"Here's how I do sleepovers"

I know a lot of kids with bedwetting avoid sleepovers, but I have found that I can do it without other people noticing. I wait until my friends are busy. Then I bring a towel, my phone, the lubricant, and the enema into the bathroom and lock the door. I hold the enema for a little less time than usual, so my friends won't get suspicious.

By the way, this is excellent news! It means you have a medical condition that can totally be fixed. With the right treatment, a stretched rectum will shrink back to its regular size and stop causing accidents.

But, there's a catch: For this to happen, your rectum must be fully cleaned out every day for several months. I'll be honest. Cleaning out the rectum is not a simple or quick process. You can't just drink capfuls of powdery medicine mixed with water and expect this pile-up of stool to dissolve and make a grand exit from your bottom. Not even high doses of powerful powders, pills, or syrups will do the job. If medications or alarms did the trick, I would not have a bedwetting clinic packed with patients!

The single most important treatment for enuresis or encopresis is a daily enema. An enema is a liquid solution you insert into your rectum, via a squeeze bottle (or bag) and a flexible plastic tube. Yes, you will be putting a tube up your butt, every day, probably for several months. I am well aware that this does not sound like fun. Yeah, it sucks. But my patients tell me that it sucks a lot less than wetting the bed or having accidents at school. They also tell me the process becomes routine. After a while, it's just not a big deal. Some of my patients even do enemas on sleepovers, and their friends are none the wiser.

When I type "enema" on my phone, autocorrect usually changes it to "enemy." But I promise you: Enemas are not your enemy! They are your ticket to dryness, though the journey may be slow.

The treatment program my patients follow is called **M.O.P.**, short for the Modified O'Regan Protocol. The protocol — a fancy word for "plan" — is named after the Irish doctor who invented it, Dr. Sean O'Regan. I tweaked his protocol a bit, which is why it's called the "Modified" O'Regan Protocol.

M.O.P. essentially has two parts: a daily enema and a daily laxative (medicine you swallow to make poop mushier or stimulate a poop). Eventually, you might combine **M.O.P.** with bedwetting medication prescribed by a doctor. But medication probably won't help unless you're also doing **M.O.P.**

M.O.P. takes commitment, patience, and experimentation, but I promise: It is not too late to fix your situation! I've worked with hundreds of bedwetting patients who were dreading college or planning to live at home instead of in a dorm. Many were seriously depressed. These kids resolved their condition on **M.O.P.**, and their lives improved greatly.

Not long ago, I received the following email from the mom of a 16-year-old. Her son was not my patient, but he followed **M.O.P.** through our books.

> ***M.O.P.*** *was literally life saving for my son, who was repeatedly hospitalized for suicidal ideation due to encopresis and enuresis. He was on board to try enemas because nothing else had worked, and we had nothing to lose. It still shocks me how much resistance we got from everyone — the GI doctor, the pediatrician, the mental health care providers, his dad. But we did it anyway, and it worked. So much ignorance from the health care system. Lots of grieving on our part once we implemented the program. My son is 16 ½ and I was finally able to buy him underwear.*

Hang in there! Help is on the way!

If you're a parent seeking support, join our private, hidden Facebook group for parents of teens and tweens. You and/or your child can post questions, and I'll be glad to answer them.

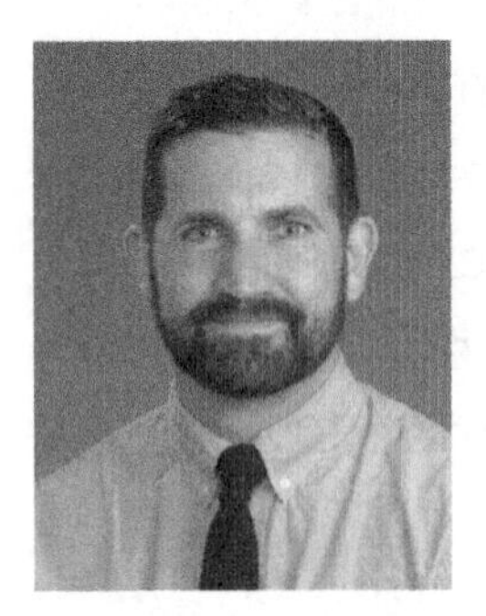

Steve Hodges, M.D.
Professor of Pediatric Urology,
Wake Forest University School of Medicine

The Language of M.O.P.

When you first hear all the words related to M.O.P. — *enema, laxative, rectum* — you may feel overwhelmed, as if you suddenly have to learn a whole new language. Don't worry: This is not like learning Spanish or Mandarin Chinese! The list of key terms is short, and there will be no tests!

You probably know some of these terms already. Scan the list, and read the definitions of any term that is not familiar. You'll get to know these terms well as you progress through M.O.P.

Anus

The opening in your butt where poop exits, aka your butthole!

Bladder

The round, stretchy organ in your body that stores pee (urine). Your bladder sits right next to your rectum (the end of your colon). When poop piles up in your rectum, the rectum stretches and presses against and aggravates your bladder. Drinking lots of water and peeing frequently helps your bladder heal.

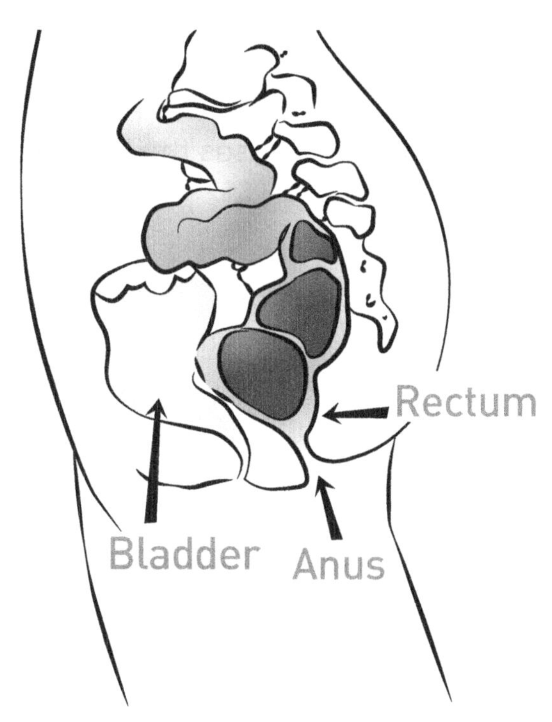

Bowel movement

Going poop, aka Number 2. Your *bowels* are your intestines, the tubular coil that connects your stomach to your anus. The waste your body can't use moves through the bowels until you poop it out. A *bowel movement*, or BM, is the act of *moving* the waste out of your bowels.

Colon

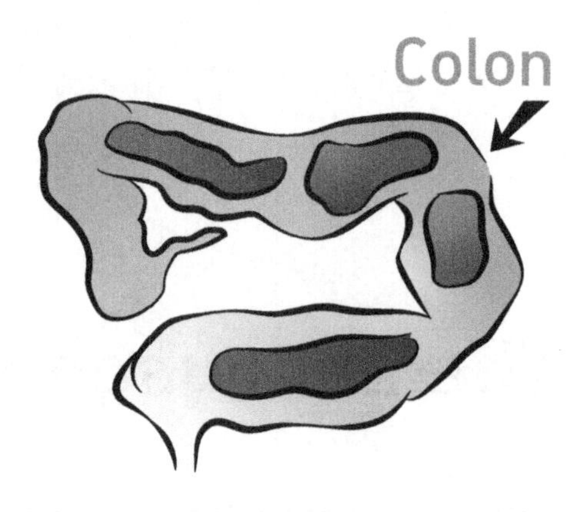

Your large intestine, the portion of your bowel designed to absorb fluid. This is where poop sometimes gets stuck, especially at the end of your colon, known as the rectum. M.O.P. is a treatment to clear out poop that has gotten stuck.

Constipation

A pile-up of poop in the rectum. This happens when you don't have a complete bowel movement every day.

Double M.O.P.

M.O.P. that involves inserting olive oil or mineral oil into your bottom through a tube. The oil sits there overnight, softening crusty old poop, and you flush it out in the morning with an enema.

Encopresis (pronounced en-coe-PREE-sis)

Poop accidents. Some adults believe kids poop in their pants on purpose, but this is false. Encopresis happens when too much stool (poop) accumulates in the rectum. This causes the rectum to stretch and weaken, so poop just falls out.

Enema

A treatment that involves inserting liquid into your anus (butthole) through a flexible tube attached to a squeeze bottle or bag. The purpose of enemas is to clear out stool that has gotten stuck in your rectum and has piled up.

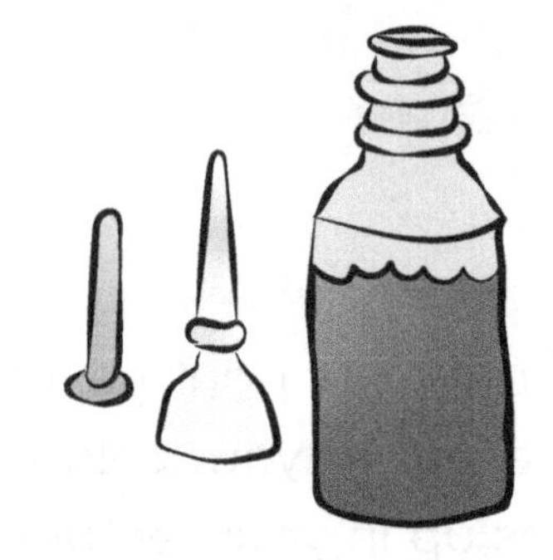

a store-bought enema

Enuresis (pronounced en-yur-EE-sis)

Pee accidents, nighttime or daytime. Both types of enuresis have the same cause: constipation. Your bladder, aggravated by a stretched rectum, empties so quickly that you have no chance of getting to the toilet on time.

Large-volume enema

An enema that stores liquid in a bag rather than a bottle. The bag holds more liquid, known as "solution," than store-bought enemas and for some kids works better than smaller enemas.

Liquid glycerin suppository, or LGS

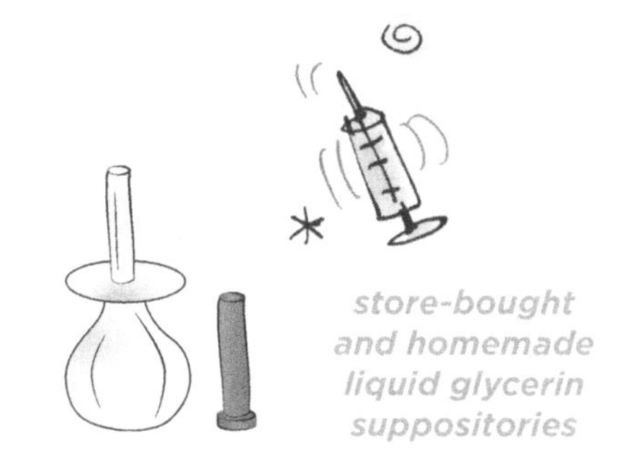

store-bought and homemade liquid glycerin suppositories

An LGS is a small enema that contains only glycerin. These can be purchased or made at home with a syringe.

M.O.P., aka Modified O'Regan Protocol

A treatment plan that resolves enuresis and encopresis. A *protocol* is simply a plan with a set of rules or guidelines. Dr. O'Regan is the Irish doctor who proved constipation causes bedwetting and developed an enema treatment plan to fix it. M.O.P. includes the word *modified* because I tweaked Dr. O'Regan's original protocol.

There are five variations of M.O.P., which use different combinations and types of enemas and laxatives. For teens and tweens, the most common versions are M.O.P.x (enemas plus stimulant laxatives) and Multi-M.O.P. (three docusate sodium mini-enemas per day, with no laxatives).

Osmotic laxative

A medication you take by mouth — in liquid, powder, or pill form — that draws water into your colon to keep poop mushy. This makes pooping less painful.

Potty sit

A 5-minute attempt to poop. I recommend this once or twice a day, ideally after breakfast and/or dinner, when your body is most primed to poop. Sitting with your feet propped on a stool helps poop exit more easily.

Rectum

The end of the colon. The rectum is designed as a "sensing" organ — when stool arrives, you're supposed to sense the urge to poop and find a toilet ASAP. But with constipation you may not feel that urge, so stool piles up in the rectum, an organ not designed for storage. Eventually, the rectum becomes floppy and loses the power to shovel out poop.

Skid marks

Poop smears in your underwear. Skid marks are a sign of constipation, not poor wiping! The smears indicate your rectum did not fully empty. "Sharts," aka messy farts or "Hershey squirts," also signal constipation.

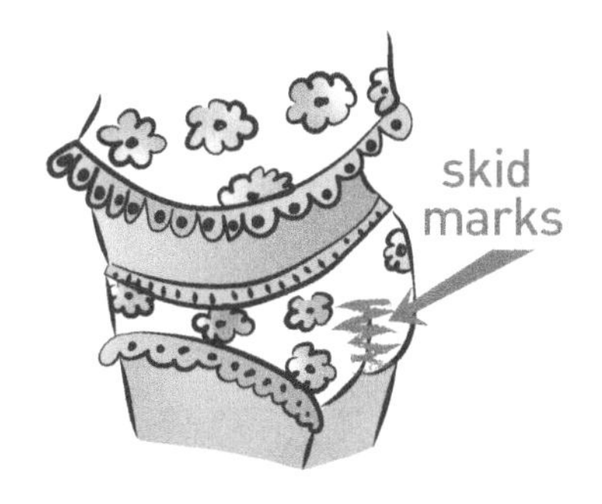

Spontaneous poop, or SP

A bowel movement you initiate yourself, without an enema. One goal of **M.O.P.** is to have a spontaneous poop every day. This may not happen at first, and you may need a stimulant laxative to help this happen. Daily SPs are a sign your stretched rectum is healing.

Stimulant laxative

A medication you take by mouth that causes you to poop. Whereas enemas trigger a bowel movement within 10 minutes, stimulant laxatives take 5 to 8 hours to kick in.

Stool

Another word for poop. Aim for a pile of mushy stool every day, like a frozen yogurt swirl or a cow patty or thin snakes. Stool that resembles a big log, turkey sausage, or rabbit pellets signals constipation.

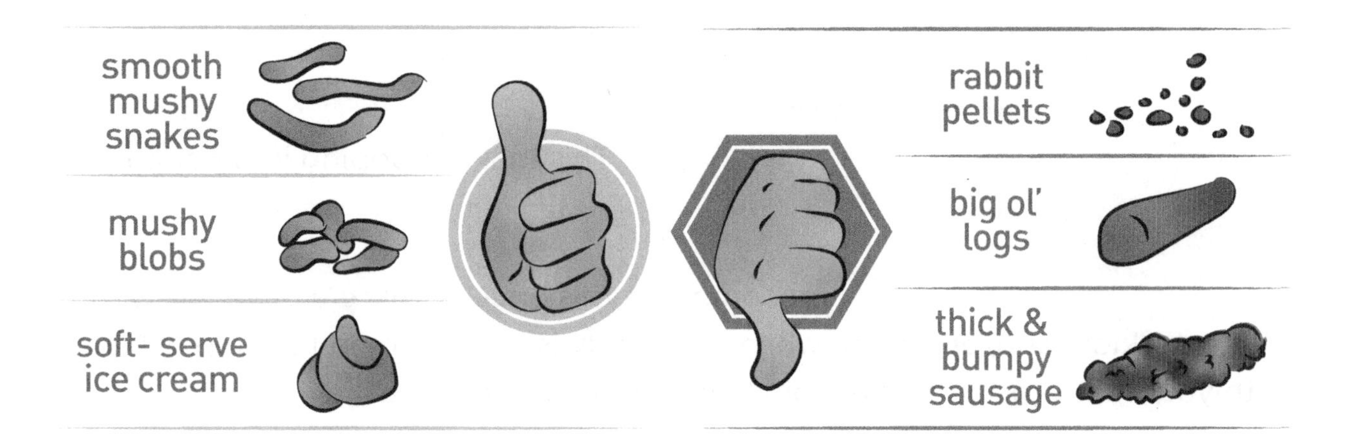

Welcome to M.O.P.

In this section, I explain the real cause of bedwetting. Spoiler alert: It has nothing to do with deep sleep!

I also answer questions that many of my teen patients ask, including: *Why didn't I outgrow accidents when other kids did? How long will it take for my accidents to stop? How did I get constipated in the first place?*

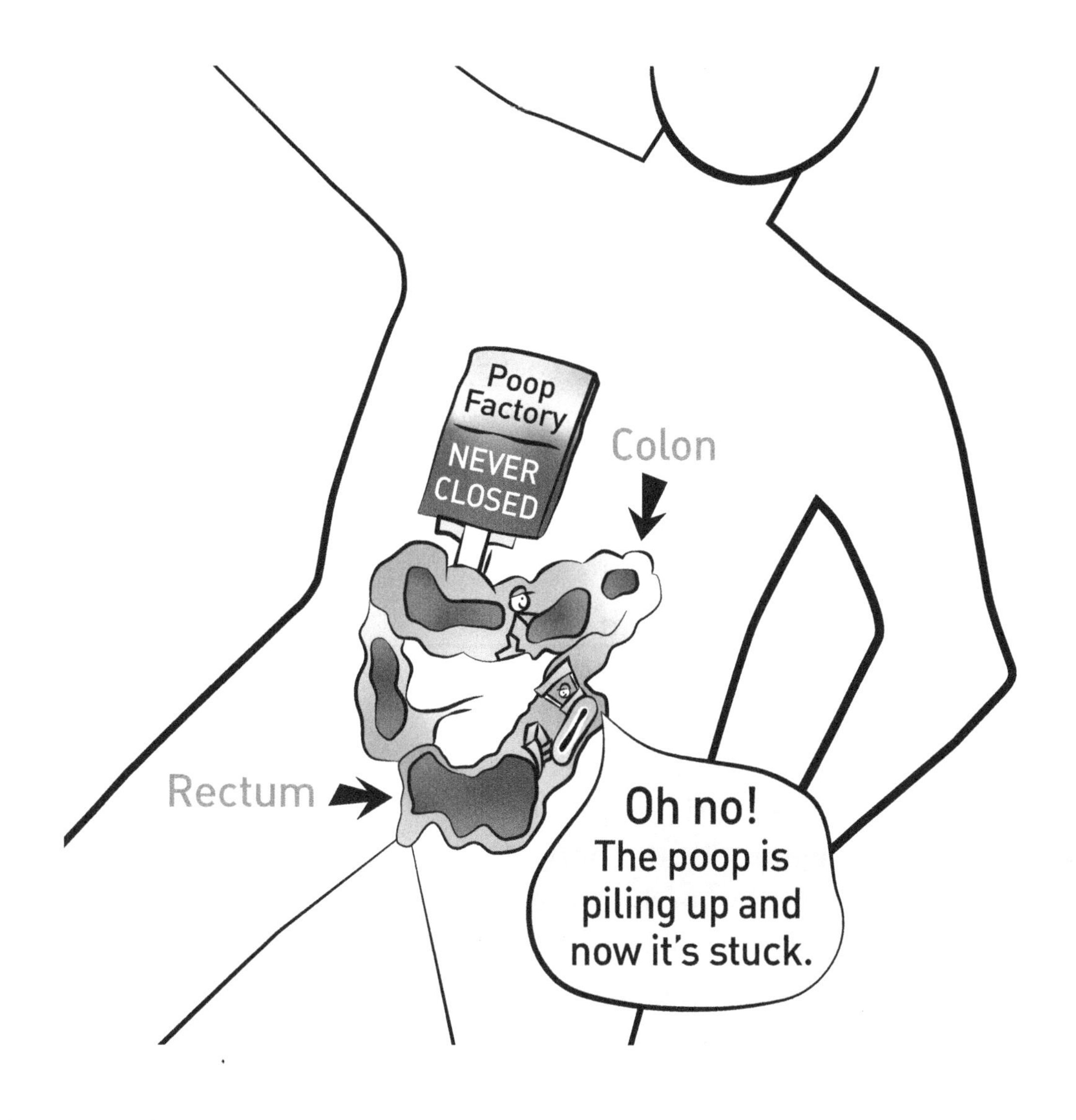

You're Getting on My Nerves — Literally: How Constipation Triggers Bedwetting (And Poop Accidents, Too)

If you're familiar with the term *constipation*, I'll bet you've heard the most common definitions: "difficulty pooping" or "having bowel movements fewer than 3 times a week." But these definitions are misleading! It's true that people who strain to poop or who poop just a few times a week are constipated. I agree with that much. However, this definition emphasizes what is *not* happening (pooping) rather than what *is* happening: poop is piling up and stretching of the rectum. That's what *I* mean by constipation. It's a much more useful definition.

So how exactly does constipation cause accidents? That's pretty simple, actually. Your rectum happens to sit next to your bladder. I mean, *right next door*. When kids are constipated for several years, as most of my patients have been, this pile-up of stool gradually stretches the rectum, so that it's a lot wider than usual. Imagine stuffing a basketball sock with a whole bunch of rolled-up socks: The more rolled-up socks you shove in there, the wider the sock will get. You get the idea!

Eventually, the stretched rectum starts to press on the bladder, aggravating the bladder nerves. Under normal circumstances, when your rectum is not stretched, your bladder nerves alert your brain that it's time to pee *only* when your bladder is full; you receive the signal, feel fullness in your bladder, and head to the toilet. But . . . when your bladder nerves are stretched by a stuffed rectum — well, your bladder overreacts. Big time. Instead of calmly alerting you that you should find a toilet sometime in the near future, your bladder goes nuts, squeezing and emptying right then and there, without bothering to inform you in advance. You can't stop an accident

You can't stop an accident from happening any more than you can stop a sneeze or a hiccup.

from happening any more than you can stop a sneeze or a hiccup. There's *no way* you have time to wake up, let alone sprint to the toilet.

About one-third of my teen and tween patients with bedwetting have daytime pee accidents, too. (Some also have poop accidents, which I'll address shortly.) Daytime accidents happen for the same reason as bedwetting: The overactive bladder squeezes too quickly and forcefully for you to get to the toilet. On M.O.P., daytime accidents usually stop before the bedwetting does.

How Poop Builds Up in the Rectum

Now let's talk about how stool piles up in the first place. You've probably learned about the digestive system in school, but let's do a quick recap. Food that you've chewed and swallowed gets mashed up by your stomach and then propelled ahead to your small intestine. There, the remains are broken down further and all the nutrients — vitamins, minerals, carbs, fats, and protein — are absorbed through your small intestine into your bloodstream. What's left over — the waste your body can't use — then gets transported to your large intestine, aka the colon. This is your body's last chance to absorb water into your bloodstream. At this point, the leftover waste becomes increasingly firm and dry as it progresses toward the exit.

Your body is a poop factory that never closes, a continual conveyor belt. If you delay pooping even by one day, you'll end up with a logjam in your rectum.

The final stop on the digestive tract is the rectum, the very end of the colon. Your rectum is designed to be a *very* temporary storage area. When stool arrives, the walls of the rectum briefly expand and nerve receptors signal your brain, which, in turn, triggers the urge to poop.

But . . . we humans have the ability to override that signal by tensing our pooping muscles. We can delay pooping for hours, even days. We are masters of delay! There are lots of reasons humans delay pooping, often without realizing it. Maybe you're in the middle of a science lab or a basketball game, or you're on an airplane. Or maybe your school bathroom is gross and you're just not comfortable pooping there, or you've had painful pooping experiences, so you automatically ignore that signal. I can think of about a million scenarios where you might think: *Eh, I'll poop later.*

There's just one problem: Your body's digestive process doesn't stop! Your body is a poop factory that never closes, a continual conveyor belt. If you delay pooping even by one day, you'll end up with a logjam in your rectum. You probably won't notice this, because your rectum has a remarkable capacity to stretch, like socks or yoga pants! But eventually, this stretching causes problems.

Bedwetting and pee accidents are two conditions caused by a stretched rectum, but they're not the only ones. Poop accidents (encopresis) and underwear "skid marks" (poop smears) can happen, too. That's because over time, a stretched rectum loses sensation and the muscle tone to push stool out the door. So, when stool arrives in your rectum, you may not receive that "Hey, it's time to poop — get your butt to the toilet!" signal. You just don't feel it at all. And even if you do, your rectum may not have the oomph to shovel all of it out your butt and into the toilet. Think about socks that have been stretched out over time: They lose their elasticity and become kind of floppy.

Many adults don't believe anyone could have a poop accident without noticing, so they assume the kid did it on purpose. But that is just totally wrong!

With some kids, poop just drops out of their bottom — with no warning, in the middle of P.E. class or at a friend's house, without the kid even feeling it. Many adults don't believe anyone could have a poop accident without noticing, so they assume the kid did it on purpose. But that is just totally wrong! No kid would ever poop in their pants intentionally. If you understand how constipation works, it's very easy to grasp why a kid could have a poop accident without feeling it.

Have you ever found skid marks in your underwear, without having a full-fledged poop accident? The same process is at work. It just means your rectum wasn't able to push out all the stool. Some got left behind and smudged your underwear. It has nothing to do with how well you wiped.

For some kids, constipation — poop piling up, the rectum stretching — causes

You can actually measure the diameter of the rectum to see whether it is stretched beyond normal size.

discomfort. They get stomachaches or feel pain when they poop. After all, the longer stool sits in your rectum, the harder, drier, and larger the pile-up becomes, so when you actually do poop, you've got to push out a big ol' log, and that can hurt. I know! I spent most of my childhood constipated and just figured pooping was something that hurt. I never mentioned my difficulties to anyone.

On the other hand, many majorly constipated kids feel no pain, not even a stomachache. Most of my patients are surprised to learn they have an enlarged rectum. Few have ever been told that a pile-up of stool can aggravate the bladder nerves.

In fact, some of my patients are so shocked by this explanation that they don't believe they are constipated. But it's easy to prove with an X-Ray of your abdomen. You can actually measure the diameter of the rectum to see whether it is stretched beyond normal size. Later in this guide, I explain how X-Rays can be helpful.

Bottom line: Virtually all cases of enuresis and 100% of encopresis cases are caused by a stretched rectum. With enuresis, I say "virtually all" because there are some medical conditions that can cause wetting. I discuss these conditions in *The M.O.P. Anthology 5th Edition*, but they are almost always diagnosed years before middle school and are highly unlikely to be causing your accidents.

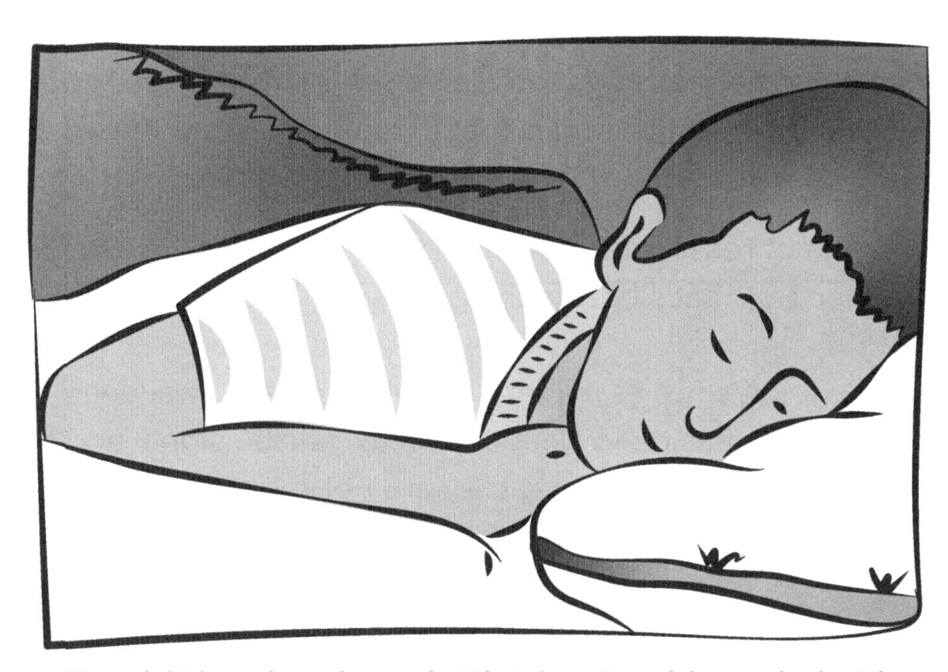

You might be a deep sleeper, but that doesn't explain your bedwetting.

Most kids have no idea that delaying pooping has consequences. I had no clue when I was a kid. So don't get down on yourself about past withholding! It's an extremely common habit and one that's within your power to reverse. Just do your best to poop in a timely manner any time that's possible. I don't expect anyone to dash off the soccer field in the middle of a game, but if you're in a class when the urge strikes, go as soon as you possibly can.

No, Deep Sleep Has Nothing to Do with Bedwetting

Virtually every high-school student who lands in my clinic has been told that "deep sleep" is the cause of their bedwetting. This is a very popular theory! The idea is that bedwetting kids sleep so soundly that they just don't feel the urge to pee. One mom told me, "I could run a vacuum next to my son's head and he would never wake up!"

That may be true, but it does not explain her son's bedwetting.

If you search the internet, you'll find loads of articles stating the "deep sleep" theory as fact. Even the American Academy of Pediatrics, a huge and influential organization of pediatricians, promotes this idea. The academy states that a "deep sleep pattern can be part of normal adolescent development, as can a poor sleep schedule and too few hours of sleep." I think what they're suggesting is that inadequate sleep makes kids super tired, which leads to deep sleep, which somehow causes bedwetting?

This line of reasoning makes no scientific sense. You may very well be a deep sleeper. But that's beside the point, because kids with typical bladders — bladders not aggravated by a stretched rectum — simply do not need to pee overnight. It's not as if light-sleeping kids are awakened overnight by the urge to pee, whereas deep sleepers fail to get the signal and therefore wet the bed. If you have siblings, I'll bet they are not regularly waking up to pee at 2 a.m. More likely, they sleep through the night and pee in the morning.

The fact is, no child, whether a light sleeper or a heavy sleeper, should even have the urge to pee at 2 a.m. Deep sleep cannot cause a bladder to go haywire and hiccup in the middle of the night. Because human beings typically

The bladder just spazzes out too quickly for you to wake up and react. So, boom: wet sheets.

don't eat or drink overnight, we don't produce enough urine to need to pee. A healthy bladder is large enough and stable enough to hold the urine we do produce.

When any person, child or adult, needs to pee overnight, it's because the bladder is overactive, spasming when it's not full. In children, this overactivity is caused by the rectum irritating the bladder. Plenty of adults, most of them over age 40, have bladder overactivity, but this is typically due to changes in the bladder that occur with age, though constipation can contribute.

Still, you are probably wondering: *Why don't I wake up in time to avoid an accident?* Because adults with an overactive bladder experience a type of spasm that is less forceful and comes on slowly enough to let them wake up and get to the toilet. Children, by contrast, experience more powerful, abrupt bladder spasms. The bladder just spazzes out too quickly for you to wake up and react. So, boom: wet sheets.

Bottom line: Most kids are deep sleepers. Most kids don't wet the bed. It doesn't matter if you could sleep through an insanely loud concert. That still can't explain why your bladder needs to empty overnight.

Over the years, you may have been given other explanations besides deep sleep, such as kidneys that produce too much urine or a bladder that's unusually small. None of these theories hold up, as I explain in detail in the *Anthology*.

The Top 7 Questions Teens Ask About Accidents

Most of my patients don't want to have long conversations about bedwetting. I get it. This is not a fun topic to discuss. But here are the questions they ask most often, in case you have the same questions on your mind.

#1. How many other teenagers have enuresis?

Most of my teenage patients think they are the only kids their age who have accidents. But that is hardly the case! About 2% of all kids age 11+ experience bedwetting — about 1 in 50 tweens and teenagers. Maybe 2% doesn't sound like a lot, but in the United States, there are about 25 million kids ages 12 to 17, so that means more than half a million of them have enuresis.[1] Probably one-third of those have daytime accidents too.

> **TEENAGE ENURESIS:**
>
> More Common Than You Think.
>
> - **500,000+ American kids ages 12 to 17 have enuresis**
> - **Enuresis is about as common as autism:**
>   - **1 in 50 teens have enuresis**
>   - **1 in 54 kids have autism**

That is a ton of kids — in fact, more teenagers have enuresis than have autism. With bedwetting, it's about 1 in 50. With autism, it's 1 in 54.[2] You hear about autism all the time, but no one ever talks about enuresis.

The average high school in the United States has about 750 students, which means there are probably 15 kids with enuresis in a typical school. In a big-city high school, with 2,000 to 4,000 students, there are probably 40 to 80 students with enuresis. Think about that next time you walk the hallways!

#2. Why didn't I outgrow this when other kids did?

You probably have plenty of friends who outgrew bedwetting or daytime accidents, even if they never talked about it. Why didn't you get so lucky?

At least 10% to 30% of kids around the world are constipated, for reasons I explain in question #3, but some kids' bladder nerves are just more sensitive when pressed on by the rectum. In other words, one child's bladder might hiccup when the rectum is only slightly stretched and barely touching the bladder, whereas another child might not experience bedwetting unless the rectum is stretched to triple the normal diameter and is crushing the bladder.

The constipated kid with the less sensitive bladder may never develop enuresis or may stop wetting with small improvements in constipation. For example, maybe the kid switches to a school with a cleaner bathroom or has a teacher

1 POP1 Child population: Number of children (in millions) ages 0–17 in the United States by age, 1950–2019 and projected 2019–2050. In ChildStats.gov. Retrieved from https://www.childstats.gov/americaschildren/tables/pop1.asp

2 Data & Statistics on Autism Spectrum Disorder. (2020, March 25). In CDC.gov. Retrieved from https://www.cdc.gov/ncbddd/autism/data.html

who's more chill about bathroom passes. There are lots of reasons kids might become less constipated over time and less prone to bedwetting. But some don't and need a treatment such as M.O.P.

Bottom line: Whether bedwetting stops sooner or later, I believe, depends on how much the rectum is stretched and how sensitive the child's bladder is to that stretch. These are just not factors you can control.

#3. How did I end up constipated in the first place?

I urge kids and parents not to dwell too much on how all this happened. Chances are, your constipation began many years ago. You're better off focusing on treatment than on what may have happened when you were 3 years old. However, I'm sure you are curious, so I will explain the most common reasons kids develop constipation.

Genetics may be the biggest factor. Some kids are just more prone to getting clogged up than others. In some families, all the kids need eye glasses; in other families, all the kids have accidents and need M.O.P.

On top of that, we live in the 21st century. In modern society, loads of kids need help pooping, for the same reason so many kids need braces: since ancient times, our lifestyle has changed, but our bodies have not kept up.

Back when humans were hunter-gatherers, our roomy jaws easily accommodated our 32 chompers. But over time, as we shifted from hunting and gathering to farming, supermarket shopping, and chewing softer foods, our jaws downsized. However, we still have 32 teeth! So, most of us need our wisdom teeth pulled by an oral surgeon and need braces to fix the rest.

In some families, all the kids need eye glasses; in other families, all the kids have accidents and need M.O.P.

A similar scenario has unfolded in our guts. Before PopTarts, couches, ipads, and toilets, constipation was rare. Humans mostly ate plants, spent most of the day active, and squatted to poop when they got the urge. But the human digestive system wasn't designed to handle processed food and our relatively slothful lifestyles. So, these days, stool moves through the digestive tract at a pokier pace. Our conveyor belts have slowed down.

That's not all! Our society's concept of decency has changed. In modern times, you can't just poop anywhere! Unless you're backpacking in the woods, you need a toilet, or you will probably get arrested. But the flush toilet itself causes problems, because it takes us out of the natural squat position. That's why I recommend pooping with your feet on a foot stool. Studies prove that poop exits much more easily in that position.

Basically, human beings are too smart for our own good. It would not occur to a cat, or to our prehistoric ancestors, to delay pooping when the urge strikes.

Basically, human beings are too smart for our own good. It would not occur to a cat, or to our prehistoric ancestors, to delay pooping when the urge strikes. But today's humans, particularly human kids, often override the signal to poop by tensing our pooping muscles. Sometimes we do this because pooping hurts. Other times, we do it because pooping is inconvenient, like when we're in a car or the middle of math class. Young kids, especially, get into the habit of delaying pooping, especially if they're shy in preschool. Maybe you were one of those kids! Or, maybe you even became constipated as a baby, before you could even walk. This is a common scenario, too, and often goes untreated because doctors don't take constipation seriously in children that young.

I can't say why any kid in particular developed constipation, but here's a closer look at three common reasons in our society. They might apply to you, or they might not!

- Our eating and exercise habits

  I have patients who are severely constipated even though they have never been to McDonald's, happily eat quinoa bowls with kale for dinner, and play three sports. You can't pin all cases of constipation on a highly processed diet and sedentary lifestyle. Definitely not! Still, our culture's eating habits and diminishing physical activity are leading culprits in the rise of constipation, among both adults and kids.

  Improving your eating habits — eating a lot more fruits and vegetables and beans and a lot less fast food — is important for keeping constipation from returning once you your accidents are resolved. But dietary changes alone won't unclog your rectum or resolve enuresis (or encopresis). And if you already have stellar eating habits, changing your diet may not help at all. I have patients who were put on gluten-free or dairy-free diets for years and years — even though they hated eating this way and the food restrictions did not help their constipation or bedwetting at all.

- The rush to potty train

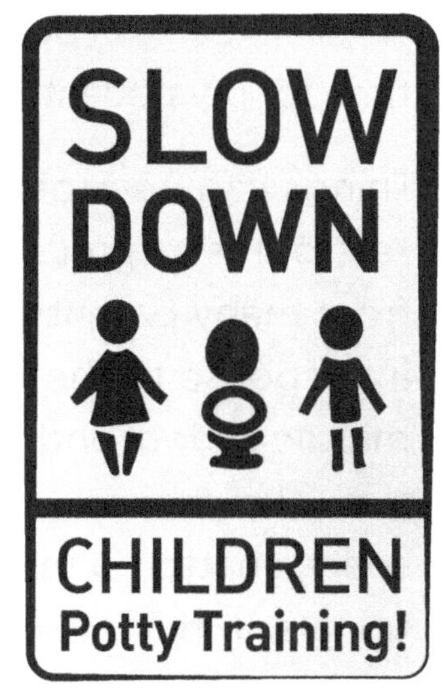

Our society practically demands that children potty train before they're ready.

In most of my patients, constipation started around the time they were potty trained. But don't blame your parents! Our culture practically demands that kids potty train before they are mature enough. There are books that promote potty training in 3 days! In 3 hours! Many preschools require children to be potty trained by age 3, which prompts parents to get a jump on things and train their children at age 1 or 2. That is too young.

Why? Because toddlers don't understand the importance of using the toilet when nature calls. They think you dash to the bathroom only when you desperately need to. At preschool these newly trained kids often feel too shy to tell the teacher they need to use the toilet. Or, they're too excited by all the fun or worried another kid will steal their toy truck while they're in the bathroom. So, they ignore the signal to poop and eventually become expert holders.

- Restrictive school policies

Many of my patients go from 7:30 a.m. to 3:30 p.m. without peeing and would never, ever poop in a school restroom. Many won't venture in there to pee, either. Some students can't get bathroom passes. Others worry they'll miss out on instruction or displease their teachers. Others are too grossed out to use school toilets. I've heard about stalls littered with toilet paper, hair-clogged sinks, and toilet water that's brown. One of my teenage patients reported "mystery smells" in her school restrooms and told me: "There were times after lunch where I felt completely bloated, and I knew I had to go to the bathroom, but I wasn't about to use it. No way."

At some schools, bathroom bullying is a problem, too. I experienced that myself. At my middle school, if you tried to poop, students would bang on the stall doors or try to open them or throw wet paper towels at you. I was terrified of setting foot in the restrooms.

You already know the consequences of withholding poop, but withholding pee also contributes to enuresis by further aggravating the bladder. It's really important to pee every 2 to 3 hours, right when the urge strikes, not 20 minutes later. But at many schools, that's just not allowed. I write notes all the time for my patients so they can use the school restroom whenever they need to.

Things can be especially difficult for my patients when schools close restrooms as punishment for poor student behavior. I received emails from many parents after dozens of U.S. schools closed their restrooms in response to the TikTok "bathroom challenge," which prompted middle school and high school students to vandalize their schools. For sure, the property damage was outrageous. Students ripped out toilet seats, shattered mirrors, clogged toilets, and attempted to unbolt urinals. In response, exasperated administrators shut down many bathrooms entirely. The mom of a high school freshman told me: "My son is angry that kids are being so stupid, but he's even more livid with the administration."

I received emails from many parents after dozens of U.S. schools closed their restrooms in response to the TikTok "bathroom challenge."

On his campus of 3,000 students, all but three restrooms closed, and students weren't allowed to use them at the beginning or end of each class period. "The administration is not considering medical needs at all," the mom told me. "They have no idea." It's true that most teachers and principals have no idea of the problems that policies like these cause for kids with enuresis and encopresis. Educators just don't receive any training on these issues.

#4. Why didn't anyone notice I was constipated?

Many of my patients want to know how they were allowed to go for so long without treatment — why year after year, doctors told them, "Don't worry, you'll outgrow it."

I don't know your situation, but I do know that 1.) some doctors don't know constipation causes enuresis, and 2.) the methods doctors are taught to detect constipation are highly unreliable. In medical school, I learned to diagnose constipation by asking families how often the child poops and feeling the child's abdomen with your hand. But this information tells you very little.

X-Rays don't lie! You can see for sure whether there is stool in the rectum.

The reality is, many kids with constipation poop every single day. But they don't fully empty, which is what matters. So, it doesn't help to know how often they poop. Sure, if you're only pooping 3 times a week, that's an obvious sign of constipation, but many of my patients poop 2 or 3 times a day. Adults think, "Oh, my kid is a great pooper!" They don't realize pooping that much signals the child is never fully emptying.

Also, when a doctor feels a child's belly, there's no way to tell if the rectum is harboring large amounts of stool. In many kids, even the skinniest kids, you just can't feel anything. That's why I X-Ray all my enuresis patients. X-Rays don't lie! You can see for sure whether there is stool in the rectum and measure how much the rectum is stretched by the pile-up.

I recently received an email from the mom of a 15-year-old who'd never had a dry night. The boy had been evaluated for constipation at age 10 and deemed not constipated. "Honestly," the mom wrote, "we don't believe constipation is the cause of his bedwetting." I suggested the boy get X-Rayed. She reported back, "Turns out his colon is full of poop!" She went on, "I am feeling a sense of disappointment that in 5 years of treatment at a major hospital, no one offered us an X-Ray." This happens all the time.

#5. How long will it take for my accidents to stop?

I wish I could give you an exact time frame and tell you it will happen fast! But that would not be honest. The truth is, resolving enuresis is not a quick fix.

On M.O.P., poop accidents actually do stop pretty quickly — usually within a few weeks, although you still have to complete the 3-month enema program to prevent the accidents from returning. But enuresis, especially nighttime enuresis, takes a lot longer to resolve than encopresis.

I can't predict how long any specific teenager will need to be on M.O.P., but I would plan on at least 6 months. By the way, this does not mean 6 months to a year of enemas every single day; at some point, you will shift to doing enemas less often and then not at all. If you try Multi-M.O.P., a variation of M.O.P. that involves three mini-enemas per day, you may be able to speed up progress somewhat.

> **"My first reaction to M.O.P. was, *What the heck?* But I had tried everything else and was feeling hopeless, so I was willing to try. I am glad I did. After two months I was having 2-3 dry nights a week. By the fourth month, it upped to 3-4 nights a week. Now I barely ever wet."**
>
> — 14-year-old on M.O.P.

But the fact is, a rectum stretched for several years won't bounce back overnight. Also, when your bladder nerves have been irritated for years, it can take months for them to settle down, even after your rectum is persistently clear. In those cases, bladder medication may help.

> **Accidents won't resolve until your rectum is fully cleaned out every day, and that can be more challenging than it sounds.**

In general, it takes about 3 months for a stretched, empty rectum to shrink back to size. But the key word is "empty." Accidents won't resolve until your rectum is fully cleaned out every day, and that can be more challenging than it sounds. You can do enemas every day for 6 months and get nowhere if the particular type of enema you are using isn't doing the job.

That's why it's so important to keep track of your progress on M.O.P. and tell a parent what's going on. You need to keep tweaking the regimen until you figure out the combination of enemas and laxatives that works for you. And this is important: "Progress" on M.O.P. does not necessarily mean dry nights at first. Even when you're still wetting the bed every night, you might start pooping more during the day, having fewer stomachaches, or feeling less urgency to pee. Sometimes the early signs of progress are not obvious.

Later in this guide I explain exactly what to keep track of. It's important to work as a team with your parents. I know reporting how often you poop or wet the bed is not fun, but if you don't track these indicators, you may end up wasting your time. That is the last thing I want for you!

My advice: Start M.O.P. expecting a long haul. You may get lucky and see dry nights in the first month, but don't give up if it takes a lot longer!

#6. Do I really have to stick an enema up my butt?

I wish I could offer you an easier way! I wish laxative powders and pills and syrups and chocolate-flavored squares would do the trick. But in most kids with enuresis or encopresis, these remedies just aren't powerful enough to clean out the rectum. Neither are weekend "clean-outs" — where you drink glass after glass of laxative powder mixed with water and spend the entire weekend pooping or waiting to poop. The problem with clean-outs, besides ruining your weekend, is that the freshly softened stool just oozes around the hard mass of accumulated stool. So, you can end up with both diarrhea and constipation! And even when oral clean-outs "work," the effect is usually just temporary.

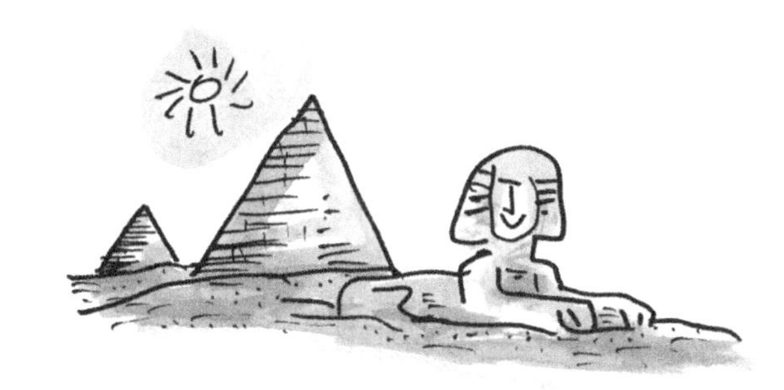

Enemas are as old as medicine. They are mentioned in Ancient Egyptian medical texts from 1500 B.C.E.

Illustration by Mark Beech

No one wants to hear this, but bottom-up treatments (sticking medication up your butt) are far superior to top-down treatments (swallowing medication). My own research confirms this. In a study of 60 kids with daytime enuresis, conducted in my clinic, some kids did M.O.P. and others used laxative powder. About 85% of the enema kids were dry within 3 months, compared to just 30% of the laxative kids. This study focused only on daytime accidents, which resolve more quickly than bedwetting, and these patients were

No one wants to hear this, but bottom-up treatments (sticking medication up your butt) are far superior to top-down treatments (swallowing medication).

ages 6 to 11, so teens can expect to be on M.O.P. longer. Still, you can see the big difference!

Most of my teen patients tell me that with some practice, enemas become easy to do. They're not as big a deal as they might seem at first. And even though this type of treatment might be new to your family, know that enemas have actually been around since ancient times! Enemas are mentioned in Ancient Egyptian medical texts from 1500 B.C.E. and were supported by Hippocrates, the famous Greek doctor, around 400 B.C.E. Despite all the new technology we have today, sometimes old remedies work best.

#7: What if M.O.P. doesn't work?

For my teenage patients, some version of M.O.P. almost always works. But I understand that accidents are worse for kids in middle school and high school than for younger kids, and if progress is slow, you may worry that your bedwetting will never stop. It will! I want you to know that there is a back-up plan for the most difficult situations: a surgical procedure call bladder Botox. Yes, this is the same Botox that celebrities have injected into their forehead to smooth over their wrinkles!

Botox can also be injected into a kid's bladder to stop the unwanted "hiccups" that cause accidents. With this surgery, you are under general anesthesia, which means you are unconscious and can't feel anything. The surgery takes about 15 minutes, and accidents usually stop within a week or so. Most kids are able to stay dry for many months, sometimes forever. The only time Botox doesn't work is when a child remains severely constipated. The poop-stuffed rectum still puts so much force on the bladder nerves that even Botox can't counteract it for long.

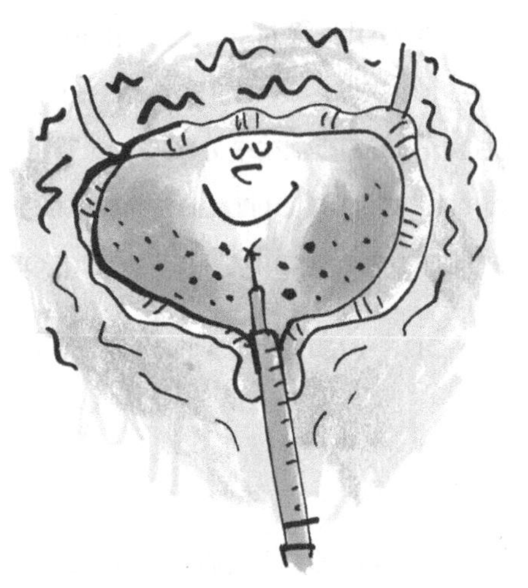

In the rare cases where M.O.P. isn't enough to stop bedwetting, injecting Botox into the bladder will fix the problem once and for all.

My enuresis patients who get the best results with Botox are the ones who have worked really hard to empty their rectum with M.O.P. and have gotten close to dryness but need help to finish the job. I'm telling you this as motivation to stick with M.O.P. and to reassure you that there is a back-up plan. I discuss bladder Botox in more detail in the *M.O.P. Anthology 5th Edition*.

SECTION 2

What's Involved in M.O.P.

In this section, I tell you about the genius doctor who invented M.O.P., a guy much smarter than me!

I also list the common signs of constipation, which many folks are not aware of. Did you know that poop smears in your underwear have nothing to do with how well you wipe your butt?

Most importantly, I explain the different products you can use with M.O.P., and the four phases of the program. You'll also hear directly from teens who have been through it.

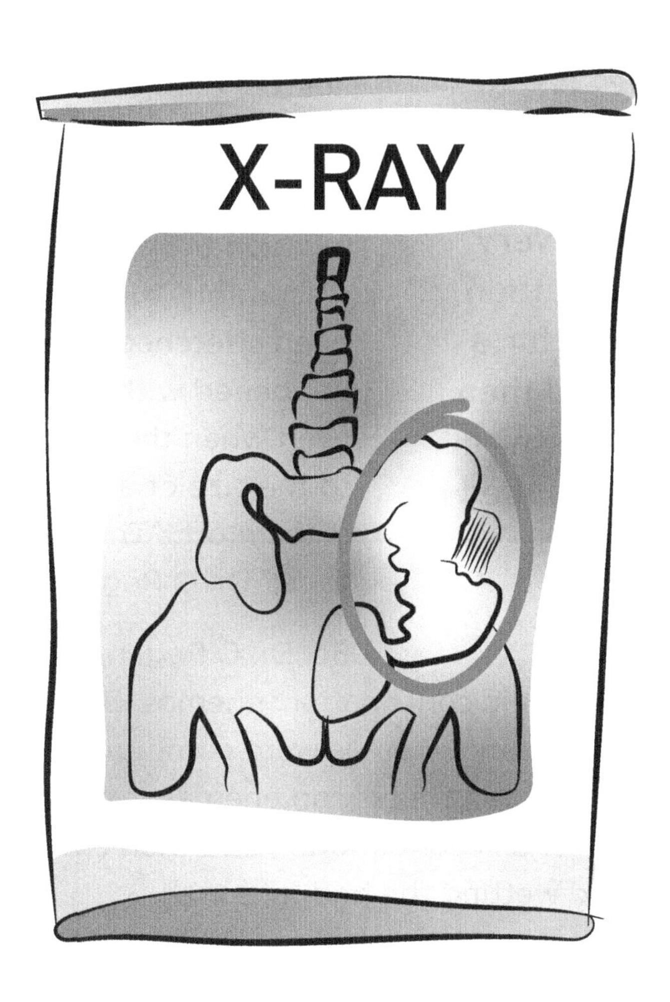

The Doctor Who Invented M.O.P.

I didn't come up with M.O.P. myself. I wish I were that smart! If you're wondering where this program came from, here's the short version of the story.

Back in the 1980s, Dr. Sean O'Regan was a kidney specialist practicing in Montreal, Canada. His 5-year-old son was wetting the bed, and Dr. O'Regan was surprised because his other two boys had stopped wetting at 3. At that time, most doctors assumed bedwetting was either a psychological issue — like, kids were doing it to get attention — or the result of a genetic abnormality in their bladder. Dr. O'Regan was not buying either explanation.

He parked himself in a library with a famous collection of European medical journals and discovered something fascinating: studies dating back to the 1890s showed a connection between constipation and enuresis. Intrigued, he asked a colleague to test his son for constipation. The colleague used anorectal manometry, a test that involves inflating a small balloon in the child's rectum. It is not a fun test, but it is highly accurate!

Dr. O'Regan gave his son enemas every night for a month, then every other night for a second month, and then twice a week for a third month. His son stopped wetting the bed.

Here's how it works: The more inflation the child can tolerate without discomfort, the more the rectum has been stretched by stool buildup. What happened with Dr. O'Regan's son? Well, even when the balloon was fully inflated, to the size of a tangerine, he felt no discomfort. "The boy's got no rectal tone," Dr. O'Regan's colleague reported.

So, Dr. O'Regan turned to the only reliable treatment for chronic constipation: enemas. Back then, laxative powders weren't available, and enemas were commonly used. No one freaked out about them! Dr. O'Regan gave his son enemas every night for a month, then every other night for a second month, and then twice a week for a third month. His son stopped wetting the bed.

After this success with his son, Dr. O'Regan and his colleague tested the program on hundreds of local children, with great success. His published studies are posted at: www.bedwettingandaccidents.com/research if you'd like to read them! I wish all doctors would read these studies. After I read them, I started X-Raying all of my enuresis patients to confirm constipation. Compared to having a balloon inserted up your butt, an X-Ray is a lot easier for kids, and it basically provides the same information. Instead of evaluating how stretchy the rectum is based on what the child feels, an X-Ray provides a clear picture of how much stool has accumulated.

In recent years, I have adjusted Dr. O'Regan's original program based on my own research and experience. For example, I have found that adding oral laxatives to enemas helps most kids. However, the standard M.O.P. program comes from Dr. O'Regan's research. Dr. O'Regan is retired now but made an amazing contribution to science. I think he is a genius!

Proving You're Constipated: X-Rays and Other Evidence

As I mentioned earlier, most of my middle-school and high-school patients are quite surprised to learn constipation is the cause of their bedwetting. They've heard so many other explanations for so long — especially the "deep sleep" theory — that they just don't believe a rectum full of poop could be causing the accidents. Most of them had no idea they were even constipated.

At least not until they got X-Rayed.

Now, a typical rectum measures about 3 cm in diameter — about 1 inch. But most of my enuresis patients have a rectum that measures at least 6 cm or 7 cm. I've had kids measure 9 cm. Sometimes on an X-Ray you can see the enlarged rectum nearly flattening the bladder. When I point this out, kids and their parents immediately understand why the child's bladder is hiccupping.

Here's an email from a mom who was shocked to learn her 17-year-old was constipated:

My daughter never demonstrated symptoms of constipation, and exams with her pediatrician have never given any indication otherwise. She was on medication for years with no success. Lots of laundry and self-confidence issues. Her X-Ray revealed her rectum measured over 7.5+ cm!

If you have no history of constipation and would like evidence that your rectum is enlarged by stool build-up, I urge you to get an X-Ray. The *M.O.P. Anthology 5th Edition* contains detailed information about ordering X-Rays and finding a doctor to properly read them. Many doctors are not experienced in evaluating X-Rays for constipation, so they can overlook a large pile of stool.

As for that 17-year-old whose rectum measured 7.5+ cm, her mom reported that after several months on **M.O.P.**, including setbacks and frustrations, the girl had success:

We are finally making progress. She has only had one accident in the last three months, has daily spontaneous poops, and is still getting a significant amount of stool with her nightly enemas. Her last X-Ray showed she was cleaned out! She leaves for college the end of August! We are so relieved to have found **M.O.P.** *just in time.*

Other Evidence of Constipation

X-Rays aren't the only way to diagnose a clogged rectum. You can figure out if you're constipated by watching for certain clues, many of which are subtle and not well known. Here are the most common red flags. Do any of them sound familiar to you?

XXL stools. I'm talking toilet cloggers! One mom reported her son's poop was the size of a Pringles can! Many folks think large poops are a good sign — I've heard people insist their child can't be constipated because she makes "big, healthy poops." But big does not equal healthy! It just means the poop has been piling up in the rectum too long.

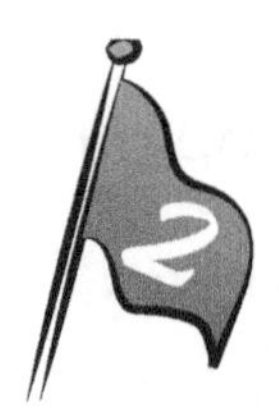

Firm stools. Poop should be a pile of mush! Like pudding or frozen yogurt or a cow patty. Thin snakes or mushy blobs are A-OK, too. But if your stool resembles a log, a turkey sausage, or rabbit pellets, you are constipated.

Infrequent pooping. As I've mentioned, you can poop every single day and still be extremely constipated. However, if you don't poop every day, then you are likely constipated. Anyone who eats every day should poop every day. It's false that some kids just "normally" poop every other day.

Pooping more than twice a day. Many folks are shocked to learn about this one. But the body is designed to poop once a day. If you're pooping 2 or 3 times a day, this means you have extra stool in the rectum just waiting to vacate.

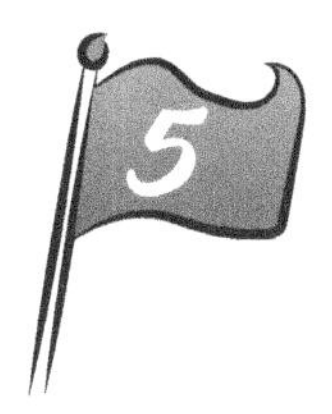

Frequent and/or urgent peeing. If you find yourself saying, "Wait, but I just peed! How can I possibly need to pee again?" you have urinary frequency. Your clogged rectum is aggravating your bladder, which is sending faulty and terribly frequent signals that it's time to pee. The same process triggers urinary urgency — the overwhelming need to pee RIGHT THIS MINUTE. On M.O.P., both frequency and urgency resolve before accidents do. That's a sign of progress.

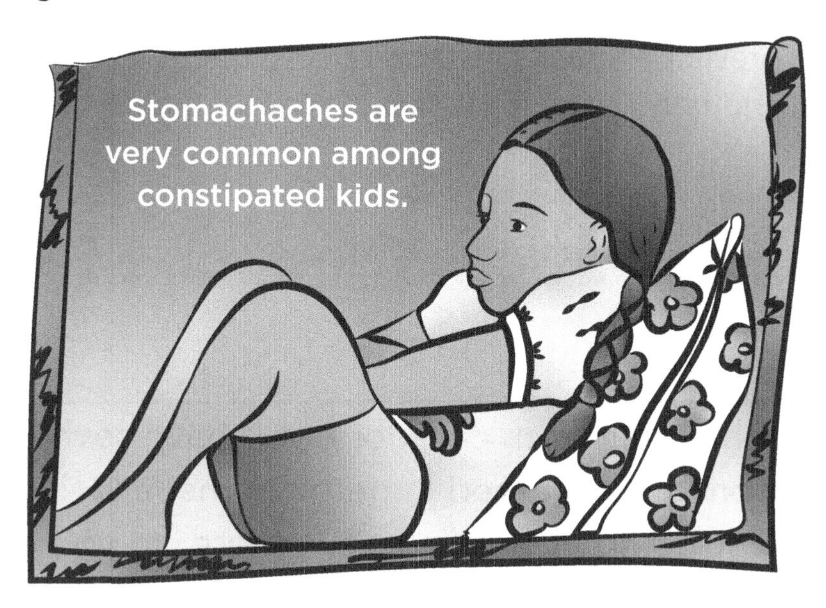

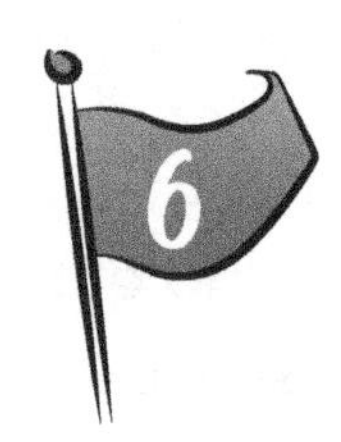

Belly pain. Many doctors dismiss belly pain in kids because the complaint is so common. But common does not mean normal! Many kids with constipation never feel pain, but kids with frequent stomachaches usually turn out to be constipated when you take an X-Ray.

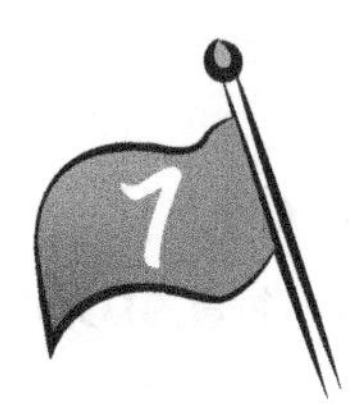

Skid marks or itchy anus. If you see poop smears on your underwear, it's not because you didn't wipe fully enough! Skid marks just mean you haven't fully emptied. If you feel the need to scratch your bottom, that's another red flag. The poop that didn't plop into the toilet is irritating the skin on your butt.

Urinary tract infections (UTIs). I have patients who get these painful bladder infections practically every month. Chronic UTIs in girls are caused by the double whammy of holding pee and holding poop. When you're harboring stool in your rectum, the infection-causing bacteria in poop are too close to the outside world. These bacteria colonize your perineum (the area between the vagina and anus) and eventually the bladder. The less often you pee, the more opportunity for the offending bacteria to crawl up to the bladder. Antibiotics will clear up an infection but won't prevent another one from taking root. A combination of **M.O.P.** and frequent peeing should clear up the problem.

The Supplies You Need for M.O.P.

Most variations of **M.O.P.** have two key components: enemas and laxatives. Within each category, you have several products to choose from, all discussed in detail in the *M.O.P. Anthology 5th Edition*. I'm including a short rundown here, so you can talk over the options with a parent. I advise experimenting with different products and brands. Some kids have strong preferences after they try a few. If one enema tip is uncomfortable for you or you don't like the taste of one laxative, try another one.

Enema Options

There are two main enema categories:

1.) stimulant enemas, which trigger a bowel movement within about 10 minutes.

2.) overnight oil enemas, which do not trigger a bowel movement but instead lubricate and soften the hard, crusty stool build-up so it washes out more easily.

Daily stimulant enemas are the most important component of **M.O.P.** Oil enemas have proven very helpful for some kids when done in addition to stimulant enemas, even just once or twice a week. Depending on how comfortable you feel with all this, you can give yourself any of these enemas, without involvement from your parents.

Here's a look at the options within each enema category.

Stimulant Enemas

Phosphate (Fleet) enema: You can buy these pre-packaged enemas at the drugstore or online. Each box contains a small bottle of saline solution (salt water) mixed with phosphate, an electrolyte that stimulates the bowel movement. (Electrolytes are chemicals in the blood that regulate our nerve and muscle function, hydration level, and blood pressure.) Phosphate enemas are a common starter enema for **M.O.P.** However, for some kids, phosphate causes an internal burning sensation, in which case I recommend switching to a glycerin-based enema.

Liquid glycerin suppository (LGS): A liquid glycerin suppository is just a small enema. The bulb containing the liquid is the size of a large grape, whereas a phosphate enema bottle is the size of a small juice glass. Liquid glycerin suppositories contain nothing but glycerin, a clear, syrupy liquid that triggers a bowel movement. You can buy pre-packaged LGS or, to save money, make them at home with a syringe and liquid glycerin. (The intructions can be found in the *M.O.P. Anthology 5th Edition*.) Liquid glycerin does not cause the burning some kids feel with phosphate and work very well for most kids.

Large-volume enema: Rather than squeeze the solution from a bottle, you buy a reusable enema kit, which includes a bag attached to a small hose. Each day, you fill the bag with saline solution and then add liquid glycerin and/or liquid

Castile soap, a cleanser made from various vegetable oils. You hang the bag about 2 feet off the floor — from a doorknob or hook, for instance. To slow the flow, you hang the bag lower; to speed up the flow, you hang it higher. Large-volume enemas generally work better for encopresis than enuresis.

Docusate sodium mini-enema (Enemeez): Docusate sodium mini-enemas are the smallest enemas and the only type of enema you can use with Multi-M.O.P., a variation that works very well for teenagers. With Multi-M.O.P., you give yourself an Enemeez three times a day until your accidents stop. After that, you drop down to do two per day, then one, and so on. Three times a day — what the heck? Yes, it sounds nuts, but it works very well and is explained in the *M.O.P. Anthology 5th Edition*.

Overnight Oil-Retention Enemas

If you don't make progress on M.O.P. in the first month or two, you might want to add periodic overnight oil enemas, using either olive oil or mineral oil. We call this Double M.O.P., because you are doing two enemas in a day, though they serve different purposes.

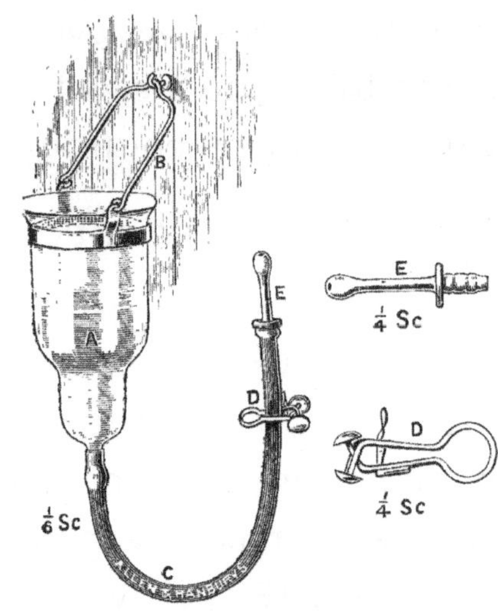

Oil enemas have been around for almost 200 years! Fortunately, today we have squeeze bottles, so you don't have to use a device like this one, used in the 19th century.

With Double M.O.P., you insert the oil enema right before bed, after you've used the toilet for the last time, and the oil stays inside you all night. In the morning, you administer the stimulant enema to flush out stool build-up and the oil. Under normal circumstances, it's difficult to do the stimulant enema in the morning rush before school, so kids usually just do Double M.O.P. on the weekends. Whether you use olive oil or mineral oil is personal preference. You can purchase pre-packaged mineral oil enemas, but you need to make your own olive oil enemas.

Laxative Options

The word *laxative* is a general term referring to medications that make pooping easier. Both enemas and oral medications can be considered laxatives, but with M.O.P., we use the term only in reference to medications you take by mouth — pills, chewable tablets, syrups, or powders mixed with water.

There are two main laxative categories:

1.) osmotic laxatives, which simply soften and lubricate stool, so pooping is less painful.

2.) stimulant laxatives, which (like enemas) actually trigger a bowel movement.

Depending on the variation of M.O.P. you are doing, you may use osmotic laxatives or stimulant laxatives. Some kids use both; others use neither. Here's a summary of the options, discussed in more detail in the *Anthology*. .

Osmotic Laxatives

Osmotic refers to medicine that brings water into the stool, making it softer and more slippery. There are four main osmotic laxatives we use with M.O.P.:

- PEG 3350: Sold as Miralax in the United States and Movicol in the U.K., this is a tasteless, odorless powder you mix with clear liquid. Studies show it is safe for children, but some parents have reported their children became moody or aggressive after taking it. If your family does not feel comfortable with PEG 3350, try one of the other choices.
- Magnesium citrate: This comes in powder, liquid, and pill forms. Some kids don't like the taste of the powder and liquid forms and prefer the pills.
- Magnesium hydroxide: The liquid version of this stuff, known as milk of magnesia, will not win any taste awards! But, it works well and is inexpensive. There's also a pill version. In addition, magnesium hydroxide comes in chewable, watermelon-flavored tablets that taste decent but are more expensive.
- Lactulose: This is a sweet syrup available only by prescription in the United States but sold over the counter in many other countries.

You can safely take more than one osmotic laxative. Some kids take one type in the morning and another in the evening.

Stimulant Laxatives

Stimulant laxatives contain senna, a plant-based substance that triggers a bowel movement. With M.O.P., the daily enema already does this job, but for some kids, especially those who aren't pooping daily except after an enema, adding an oral version is a game changer.

The difference is that enemas stimulate a bowel movement within 10 or 20 minutes, whereas stimulant laxatives usually take 5 to 8 hours to work, so it's harder to get the timing right. You don't want the laxative to kick in while you're in the middle of math class. I recommend experimenting on a weekend rather than a school day, so you are near a toilet when you feel that urge to poop. Chocolate Ex-Lax squares are the most popular stimulant laxative used with M.O.P., but there are liquid and pill forms, too.

Heads up: Stimulant laxatives can cause cramping. I don't want anyone to feel miserable on M.O.P. but some discomfort may be necessary to stimulate that bowel movement. If you feel too much cramping, you might prefer Multi-M.O.P., a varation that replaces a stimulant laxative with an extra enema or two.

The 4 Phases of Standard M.O.P.

In this section, I will explain the basics of Standard M.O.P., the plan many kids start with. However, with teens and tweens, I often recommend starting with M.O.P.x or Multi-M.O.P., discussed in Section 3. I suggest going over the options with a parent before you choose a plan. The most important advice I can give you about M.O.P. is this: Complete all phases of the program. Don't be in a hurry! Here's an overview of the four phases.

TIP FROM A TEEN:

"Don't stop enemas before you're ready"

After 8 months, I got overexcited and stopped the enemas. I started wetting again and was angry at myself and discouraged. I asked my mom, 'Have I ruined all my progress?' What motivated me to start again was remembering how good it feels to wake up dry, with no sheets to wash, just relaxing in bed.

Phase 1:
Daily enema + daily osmotic laxative

During Phase 1, you'll give yourself one enema or liquid glycerin suppository (LGS) per day while taking an osmotic laxative daily. This phase lasts until you have completed at least 30 days of enemas AND have remained accident free for at least 7 consecutive days and nights. Be prepared: Phase 1 is likely to last much longer than 30 days.

NOTE: If you have encopresis (with or without enuresis), you won't start the daily osmotic laxative until at least week 3. In kids with encopresis, laxatives can sometimes make poop accidents worse at first.

Some kids extend Phase 1 for an extra few weeks after 7 nights of dryness, to lower the odds of accidents returning. Some kids taper to 2 nights of enemas/1 night off, or even 3 nights on/1 night off, before shifting to every other day. This is called the Slow Taper and is explained in the *M.O.P. Anthology 5th Edition*.

If you see little or no progress during the first 30 days. on any **M.O.P.** plan, you'll need to tweak the regimen. There's always something new to try, and rest assured, one of the variations will work!

Phase 2:
Enema every other day + daily osmotic laxative

Once you've completed at least 30 consecutive days of enemas and have achieved at least 7 consecutive days and nights accident-free, you are ready to start tapering. Remember, you might not graduate to Phase 2 for several months. During Phase 2, you will have an enema or liquid glycerin suppository (LGS) every other day while taking an osmotic laxative daily. If you aren't pooping every day on your own, in addition to after the enema (what we call a *spontaneous poop*), consider adding a daily stimulant laxative to your program. That's the **M.O.P.x** program.

Know that shifting to Phase 2 is a common point when accidents can come back. If you do have an accident at this point, I recommend going back to the beginning of Phase 1. This can be super frustrating and discouraging, but also the best approach if your goal is to get dry for good.

Phase 3:
Enemas twice a week + daily osmotic laxative

Once you've made it through an accident-free month with enemas every other day, you're ready to move to Phase 3: an enema twice a week, along with daily laxatives. Again, if you still aren't having a daily spontaneous poop, a stimulant laxative will help. Many kids choose to keep using enemas periodically, on any day they don't poop, to minimize the odds that accidents will come back.

The shift to Phase 3 is another common point when accidents return, which comes as a surprise and big disappointment to many kids. If you've gotten this far, you might assume you're home free, but often it just doesn't work out that way. Again, if you have an accident, even just once, return to Phase 1 and complete the phase in its entirety. Throughout Phase 3, you should be pooping every day on your own.

Phase 4:
Daily osmotic laxative — no enemas!

In Phase 4, you are done with enemas. Awesome! But . . . it's possible the accidents will come back. In my experience, continuing with a daily osmotic laxative for at least 6 months will greatly increase your odds of staying accident-free. You might also want to give yourself an enema or take a stimulant laxative on any day you don't poop.

Of course, laxatives are not a lifetime solution. The ultimate goal is for you to poop every day, on your own, without any help from enemas or laxatives. So, I suggest a gradual taper. After 6 months on Phase 4, you might start a 6-week taper. For example:

- Weeks 1 and 2: half a dose every day
- Weeks 3 and 4: half a dose every other day
- Weeks 5 and 6: half a dose twice a week

If you have been taking a stimulant laxative daily or every other day, taper similarly. Congratulations. You are done!!

Spontaneous Poop: An Important Term

With my patients, I talk a lot about the *spontaneous poop*. By this I mean a bowel movement that happens "spontaneously" — without being triggered by an enema. Of course, the main goal of **M.O.P.** is for accidents to stop. But a secondary goal is for you to feel the urge to poop every day and initiate the trip to the toilet on your own, not just after an enema.

So, yes, I'm asking you to poop twice a day! You might think pooping once a day is enough — after an enema, how much more poop could be stuck in there? Trust me — tons more! My patients who achieve dryness without a spontaneous poop are more likely to have accidents start up again. And kids who poop twice a day during the early phases of M.O.P. typically overcome their accidents faster than kids who only poop once a day. It's hard to make a dent in that big poop pile-up without pooping twice a day.

Eventually, when your rectum has healed and you're done with enemas, you'll poop just once a day, but for now, you have enough poop piled up in your rectum to poop twice, and it's important to clean out as much as you can.

Most kids do not have a daily spontaneous poop when they begin M.O.P. That is normal! When you start pooping spontaneously, that's a sign your rectum is shrinking back to size and healing. It often means you'll start to have fewer accidents soon, even if total dryness is a ways off.

If you've been on M.O.P. a month and are not having spontaneous poops, talk to a parent about using a stimulant laxative to help trigger that additional bowel movement (M.O.P.x). Or, switch to Multi-M.O.P., the program that involves two or three mini-enemas per day. Many teens prefer Multi-M.O.P. because you are guaranteed to poop at least twice a day and you don't have to take laxatives. It's a faster way to clear out your rectum.

What It's Like to Be On M.O.P.

Now that you've read what M.O.P. is all about, you may be wondering: *How much is this going to suck?*

I guess the answer is: compared to what? Giving yourself a daily enema is no one's idea of fun, but most of my teen and tween patients tell me that it's a lot better than wetting the bed every night with no end in sight. Even before they start having dry nights, they feel like they are at least working toward a goal. And when the dry nights start happening, they are pretty thrilled.

"So many kids our age are going through the same thing. I was there not long ago! As time goes on, M.O.P. gets easier, so stay positive."

— Erin, age 19

Some kids are eager to try a new treatment, since nothing they tried before has worked. They want to try M.O.P. the first day they hear about it. But most kids, understandably, aren't ready to jump right in. I suggest you take your time and think it over. Hold off until you are committed, because doing M.O.P. half-heartedly — like doing enemas every other day instead of every day — is unlikely to work.

Some kids have started M.O.P. more than once because the first time around, they weren't ready. One mom wrote:

TIP FROM A TEEN:

"It will get easier."

I'm 19 and have struggled with bedwetting my whole life. No one had a solution. When my mom told me about M.O.P., I was nervous about trying it, but I can honestly say that it has been so worth it. I've been dry for 6 months now. Keep an open mind, and give this regimen your all!

We tried M.O.P. when our daughter was in 3rd grade, and she protested. Now she's 11, and it's just part of her regular routine. She is motivated to be in it for the long haul if that's what it takes.

Sometimes, kids are more on board than their parents! As the mom of one teen wrote:

Our daughter was scared, but willing. After a few months, my husband said, "Stop the madness!" and our daughter defended the enemas. She said, "Dad! The enemas are helping me! Needless to say, he was quieted and left the room.

Many kids are motivated to stick with M.O.P. because it's the first treatment that has worked. One mom told me that after 30 days on Multi-M.O.P., her 12-year-old had 9 dry nights, the first dry nights in her life. "Her confidence is soaring," this mom wrote. This girl had taken Miralax for 5 years and had missed many camps and sleepovers. She has become such a pro that she gives herself enemas on the toilet at school. Her mom said, "She does not seem to mind. She is a determined girl."

You might feel some discomfort at first. When you're super constipated, enemas can make you feel nauseous. A few kids even throw up. But the discomfort goes away quickly as you empty out. You shouldn't have more than a few days of nausea. If you do, try a different type of enema. Never persist with any treatment that is painful.

Q&A with a 14-Year-Old on Multi-M.O.P.

"Going on sleepovers was not a big deal."

Below, a mom interviewed her son for me about his experience on Multi-M.O.P. The boy wasn't seeing enough dry night on M.O.P., so he agreed to try Enemeez enemas twice a day, once before school and once before bed. At the same time, he took desmopressin, a bedwetting medication. Once a week, as an experiment, he would skip desmopressin to see if he still needed it. Eventually, he was able to stay dry without the medication and then started tapering from the enemas.

Q: When your mom first told you about the twice-a-day plan, what was your reaction?

A: I felt a mix of "No way" and "OK." I felt like it would be really hard, but I pushed myself because I wanted to be cured. Seeing the X-Ray of my insides and understanding the treatment helped me a lot to keep me going. It ended up being much easier than I thought it would be, and after a few weeks of practice, it wasn't even a big deal to go on a sleepover or an overnight school trip in a hotel.

Q: What did you think of two enemas per day compared to one enema per day plus Ex-Lax?

A: Even though it's never fun to put something up my butt, I preferred two mini-enemas a day over Ex-Lax because I had much more control over when I was going to poop. I hate pooping at school, and a few times the Ex-Lax would kick in early, which meant I had to go poop at school. With the two-a-day program, I always knew when I was going to poop.

Q: How did you manage Multi-M.O.P. on sleepovers?

A: Going on sleepovers was not a big deal. No one seemed to notice how much time I was in the bathroom. I'd say I was pooping or do it when I was going to also take a shower. I had a toiletry kit with a zippered pocket where I'd keep the enemas and another pocket with a Ziploc bag to put in the trash when I was done, so no one would ask what I had left in the bathroom trash can.

Q: What is your best advice for teens who feel too discouraged to try enemas twice a day?

A: Just do it. It's not a big deal and it cured me.

Two Teen Siblings on 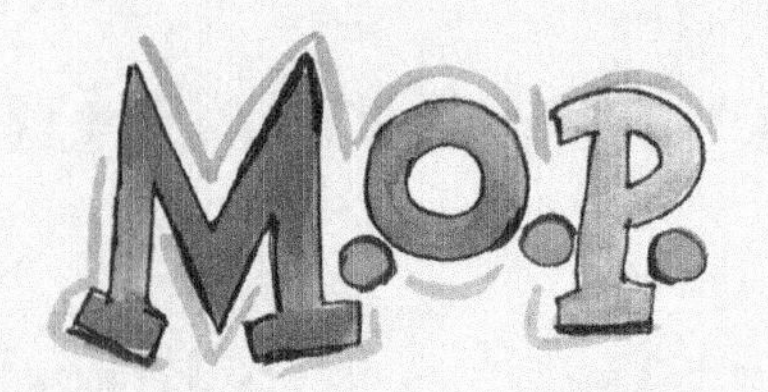 Two Different Regimens

Here's a report from a mom with two teenagers on M.O.P. Overall, it took one year for each of the teens to get completely dry. During that time, both teens needed to adjust the type of enemas and laxatives they used, the stimulant doses, and the time of day they took their medications.

The son, age 13

His enemas

Fleet phosphate enemas have always worked best for him. We tried adding mineral oil enemas, which never got much out. Neither did large-volume enemas, so we went back to Fleet phosphate. Now that he has been dry for two months, we only do the enemas on nights when he has no spontaneous bowel movement.

His laxatives

We started with lactulose in the morning, which worked well until he got really gassy. Then we switched to magnesium citrate powder with senna, which has worked well.

The daughter, age 15

Her enemas

Fleet phosphate enemas weren't producing output, so we switched to liquid glycerin suppositories. For her, adding mineral oil enemas was very helpful, and we did one a week for a while.

Her laxatives

She started on 10 ml of lactulose, which we upped to 12 ml, 15 ml, and then 20 ml before switching to magnesium citrate. That didn't have any effect no matter what dose we tried, so we switched to 30 mg of senna, which works well. On daily senna we saw the biggest improvement. Now she has been dry for 6 weeks, taking only senna and a weekly LGS just to check!

SECTION 3

Getting Started on M.O.P.

In this section, we get down to the details: How to give yourself an enema, with tips from teens who have tons of experience.

Also, you'll find a simple chart you can use to track your progress. Tracking is super important. One of the key rules of M.O.P. is: If you don't see improvement within any 30-day period, you need to tweak the protocol. I don't want you to waste time on any variation that isn't working for you!

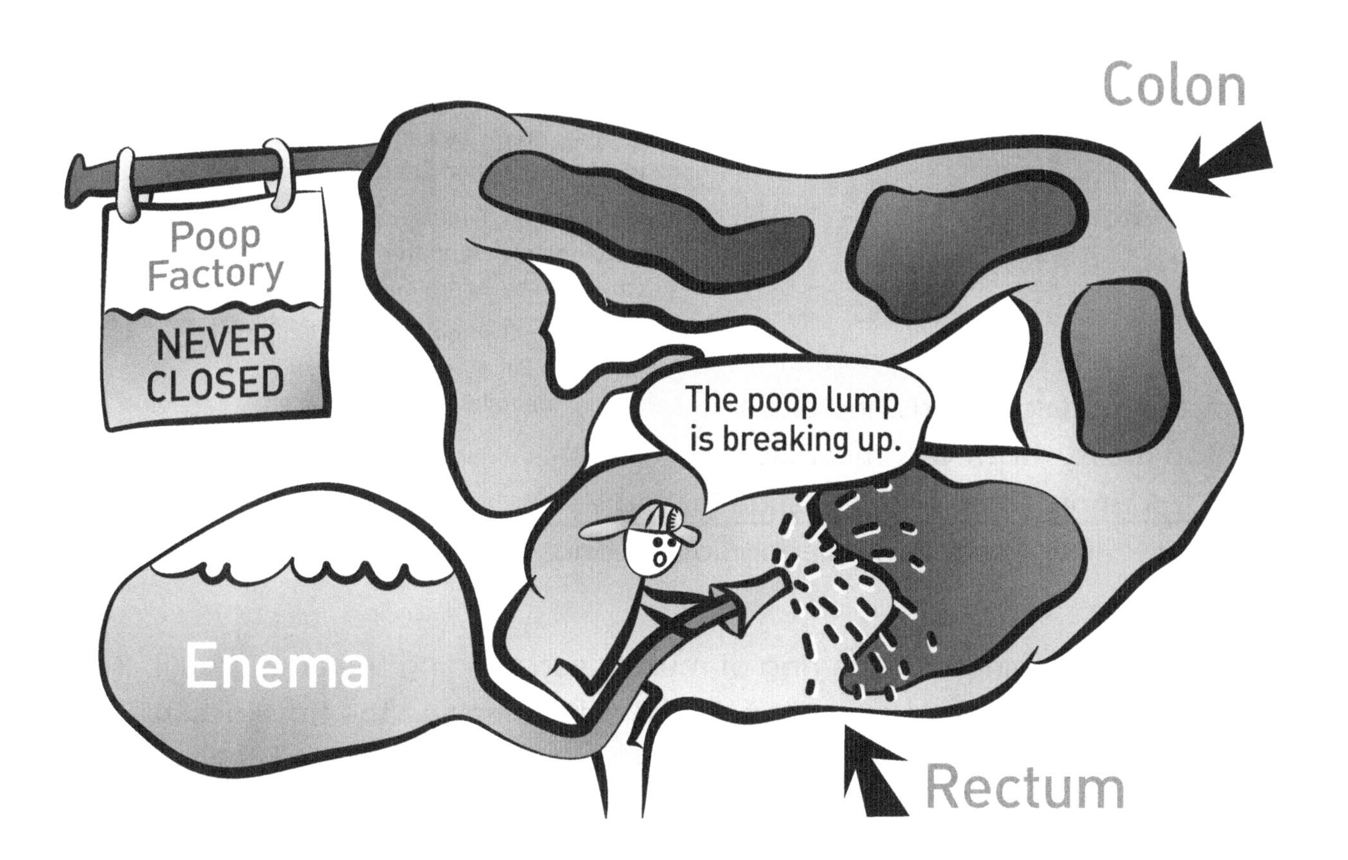

How to Give Yourself an Enema

Most of my middle-school and high-school patients prefer to insert the enema themselves, rather than have a parent do it. This way, you have privacy and control over the insertion. If you're doing large-volume enemas, which involve a reusable enema kit, you may or may not want help preparing the enema.

How to Give Yourself a Store-Bought Enema

Wash your hands before you remove the enema from the box. Then follow these steps.

Step 1: Place a towel on the floor or bed, and lie on your left side, knees bent toward your chest, aiming for your belly button. Because of the colon's anatomy, lying on your left side helps the emptying process and feels more comfortable.

Step 2: Rub lubricant on the enema tip and on your anus, aka your butthole. This is optional, as the enema tip comes lubricated, and some kids find extra lube too messy. However, most kids like to add more to help the tip slide in. You can use KY Jelly, Vaseline, Aquaphor, or coconut oil.

TIP FROM A TEEN:

"Here's how I do it:"

- First, I apply lubricant to the tip, so it doesn't hurt.
- To give myself the enema, I have found that lying on your left side takes away a lot of the discomfort.
- I place a towel on my bed, and when all the liquid has gone in, I lie on my bed until I feel the urge to poop.
- While I'm waiting, I usually watch Youtube, Netflix, or TikTok on my computer or phone, to distract me from boredom and any discomfort.
- I usually hold the liquid in for 10 to 20 minutes, and then I use the toilet, with my legs up on a stool.

Step 3: Insert the tip straight into your bottom, making sure it gets past your sphincter. The sphincter is the ring of muscle surrounding the anus. You'll know you're in when you pass the point of resistance and the tip slides in easily. This process will feel more comfortable if you are relaxed, so take deep breaths or blow out, as if you're blowing out birthday candles or blowing up a balloon.

Step 4: Squeeze the bottle slowly and steadily until you have emptied the liquid. Enema bottles have a one-way valve, so you can release and squeeze again to make sure you've emptied all the liquid. If you're extremely clogged, the enema liquid may stretch your rectum enough that it hurts; if this happens, just stop to poop. Each day, as you get more stool out, the process will become more comfortable.

Step 5: When nearly all the solution has been flushed into your rectum, remove the tube. You can sit on the toilet or lie down on the floor or on your bed until you feel the urge to poop. Aim to hold in the solution for 5 to 10 minutes, but don't worry if you have trouble holding for more than a minute or two. Once you start pooping, sit on the toilet for 10 to 15 minutes. Yes, that's a long time, but it can take a while to completely empty. Even if you feel finished, there may be more stool on the way.

How to Give Yourself a Large-Volume Enema

Giving yourself a large-volume enema is not a whole lot different from self-administering a store-bought enema but may take some practice. I recommend doing it on the floor near the toilet. You'll need to find a way to hang the enema bag about 2 feet above you, such as affixing a hook to the wall or using a hook hanging from a doorknob or towel rack.

The following instructions assume you and/or a parent have already mixed the solution (saline solution plus liquid stimulant) and poured it into the enema bag, as explained in the Anthology. If you'd like more instructions, you can find videos online by searching "how to give yourself an enema."

Step 1: Place a towel on the floor or bed.

Step 2: Lubricate the tip of the tube as well as your anus.

Step 3: Attach the hose to the enema bag, hang the bag about 2 feet above the floor. Holding the nozzle, lie on your left side, knees bent toward your chest.

Step 4: Gently insert the nozzle into your anus as deeply as you can. Take slow, deep breaths to help relax your sphincter and make the process more comfortable. If you feel cramping as the solution enters your colon, next time slow the flow by lowering the enema bag.

Step 5: When all the solution has entered your colon, remove the hose. Aim to hold the fluid for 5 to 10 minutes before pooping, but don't stress if you can only last a minute or two. Holding will get easier with time. When the urge to poop kicks in, sit on the toilet for 10 to 15 minutes. Clean the nozzle with soap and water or rubbing alcohol after each use.

Alternative M.O.P. Variations

As a middle-school or high-school student, you are probably eager for the bedwetting and/or daytime accidents to stop ASAP. For this reason, many of my patients shift to the alternative versions of M.O.P. pretty quickly or even start with one of the other options. Here's a summary of the choices. It is important for you and a parent to read the complete instructions in the *M.O.P. Anthology 5th Edition*.

M.O.P.x: Like STANDARD M.O.P., this version involves one daily enema. However, instead of an osmotic laxative, you take a stimulant laxative, so that you're guaranteed to poop twice a day. With M.O.P.x, you use a small enemas, such as Fleet or a liquid glycerin suppository (homemade or store-bought). M.O.P.x is a great place to start for kids who don't already poop every day.

MULTI-M.O.P.: This is the newest M.O.P. variation and is very simple: You give yourself a docusate sodium mini-enema (Enemeez) three times a day until all accidents have stopped, day and night. Many kids prefer this regimen to M.O.P.x because they don't have to take stimulant laxatives (like Ex-Lax). This means no cramping or nausea and no waiting around wondering when the Ex-Lax will kick in! On the other hand, it can be difficult to find the time for three enemas per day. Some kids do three enemas on weekends and two on school days. MULTI-M.O.P. must be done with Enemeez enemas, for reasons explained in the *Anthology*.

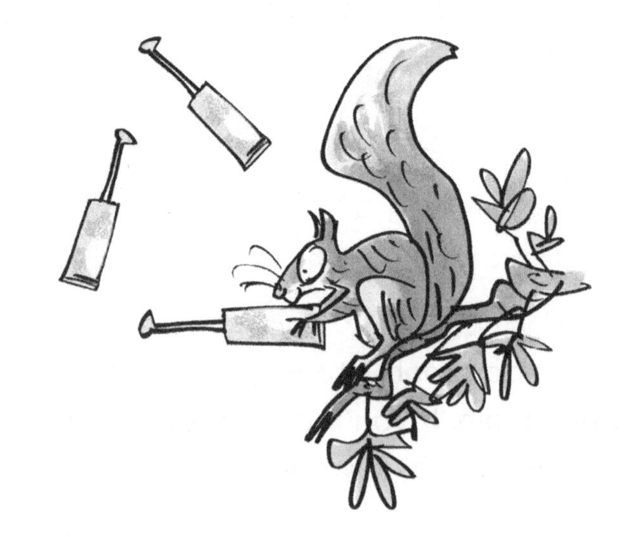

MULTI-M.O.P. involves three docusate sodium mini-enemas per day and works very well for teens.

M.O.P.+: This is the STANDARD M.O.P. program using large-volume enemas instead of small enemas. The extra volume helps many kids empty more fully. Plus, you can easily adjust the amount of stimulant to add to the saline solution. The downside is, for some kids with bedwetting, the larger volume can keep the rectum stretched, preventing healing. I recommend M.O.P.+ more for encopresis than enuresis.

DOUBLE M.O.P.: This variation calls for two enemas per day: one stimulant enema and one overnight oil enema. You do your stimulant enema in the morning, to flush out the oil that has stayed inside your rectum all night, softening the crusty old stool. Yes, this option is annoying, but it helps a lot of my patients.

Tracking Your Progress on M.O.P.

I'm sure you have plenty in your life to keep track of, including classwork, homework, and after-school activities. I don't want to pile on more work! But, taking a minute each day to track M.O.P. can save you time in the long run. You and a parent can see what's working and what's not and use that information to adjust your program to get faster results.

You can keep notes on your computer or print out one of the old-school calendars included in this guide. The MULTI-M.O.P. calendar is designed specifically for that version, and the other calendar can be used for all other M.O.P. plans. Share your log with a parent every week. Definitely don't go more than 30 days without analyzing your progress. Sometimes parents will tell me, "My kid did M.O.P. for 4 months and it didn't work." When I ask questions, I learn the family never tweaked the program the entire time! An important rule of M.O.P. is: Do not stick with any variation for more than 30 days if you are not making progress!

Signs of progress on M.O.P.

Dry nights aren't the only sign of progress on M.O.P. Before you start having fewer accidents, you will probably experience more subtle signs of progress, such as those listed below.

- fewer stomachaches
- less frequent need to pee
- less urgency to pee
- fewer underwear skid marks
- improved ability to sense the urge to poop
- more spontaneous pooping

Here's what can be helpful to track:

- Your daily enema. Check it off to make sure you did it. You might note how much you pooped, especially if you're trying a new type of enema.
- Your daily laxatives, including the dose. For example: "4 Ex-Lax squares" or "1 cap of Miralax."
- Whether you had a spontaneous poop. Our tracking chart abbreviates this as SP and includes a box to check off.
- Dry nights and/or dry days. Often kids focus on wet nights and don't realize, for example, they've gone from 5 dry nights/month to 10. That's progress!
- Other notes. Write down anything that seems important, such as whether a new laxative or enema increased how much you pooped.

Final M.O.P. Tips

I applaud all middle-school and high-school students for starting — and sticking with — M.O.P. I know the program is uncomfortable and sucks up time, and the slow pace of progress can be frustrating. It's unfair that you have to do this and your friends don't. (Of course, maybe they actually do need M.O.P. but just haven't found out about it!) At any rate, I've been working with this approach for about 15 years, and my experience and research tell me it works far better than any other method.

TIP FROM A TEEN:

"You have to be all in."

I had about 8 days dry and then decided to try a break from an enema for a night. I then had a wet night, and it made me realize that you have to keep going!

Here are a few final tips:

- Don't skip your daily enemas or laxatives. I've worked with several frustrated parents who didn't understand why their child was suddenly backsliding, only to learn the child had stopped enemas but didn't tell their parents. If you skip any part of the program, but especially enemas, it will take you longer to start seeing dry nights.

- Pee at school! I realize no one wants to use the school restroom, but peeing every 2 to 3 hours is really important for overcoming bedwetting. Your bladder is healthiest when it is filling and emptying on a regular basis. Holding your pee will only aggravate your bladder further, leading to more accidents.

TIP
FROM A TEEN:

"Communicate with your parents"

Talking to my parents was weird at first but helped a lot because they were able to make helpful changes in the program based off what I told them. A simple check-in in the morning is all you need to do.

- Keep track of your progress. Tracking M.O.P. takes less than 1 minute per day and will keep you from wasting time with products that don't work for you! Keep track digitally or print out the chart in this guide.

- Keep your parents informed. No teenager wants to share pooping details with Mom or Dad — I get that! But communication is really important, because you need to adjust the program every 30 days if you're not making progress.

It's harder to evaluate what needs to change if you keep that information to yourself. Let your parents know about dry and wet nights and whether you think the enemas and laxatives are helping you poop. If you don't feel like personally discussing it with them, just hand over your tracking sheet. Enough said!

TIP
FROM A TEEN:

"Don't be afraid to drink water at night."

I spent years trying not to drink anything after 5 p.m. When I started M.O.P., I realized drinking water actually helps you overcome bedwetting.

- Drink plenty of water. Many of my patients are afraid to drink much water because they assume that will lead to more accidents. But the opposite is true: Restricting liquids actually aggravates your bladder. One mom reported that her teenage son's soccer coach asked the whole team to drink

1 gallon of water per day. This mom and her son both worried all that water would trigger more bedwetting. But it didn't! All it did was promote more peeing during the day. Overnight, he stayed dry.

- **Expect slow progress**. Kids understandably get discouraged when a treatment that seems as extreme as M.O.P. does not bring instant results. But if you go in expecting setbacks and slow progress, you will save yourself from a lot of disappointment.

If any variation of M.O.P. doesn't help, try something new. If one formula doesn't work, keep experimenting until you find the one that does.

Stick with it, and this episode in your life *will* end!

30-Day M.O.P. Tracker

MONTHLY TOTALS:
Dry nights ____ Wet nights ____

<table>
<tr><td>DAY/DATE: ______
Enema ☐ Laxative ☐
Overnight: Wet ☐ Dry ☐
Daytime: SP ☐ Accidents ☐ ☐
NOTES: ______
______</td><td>DAY/DATE: ______
Enema ☐ Laxative ☐
Overnight: Wet ☐ Dry ☐
Daytime: SP ☐ Accidents ☐ ☐
NOTES: ______
______</td><td>DAY/DATE: ______
Enema ☐ Laxative ☐
Overnight: Wet ☐ Dry ☐
Daytime: SP ☐ Accidents ☐ ☐
NOTES: ______
______</td><td>DAY/DATE: ______
Enema ☐ Laxative ☐
Overnight: Wet ☐ Dry ☐
Daytime: SP ☐ Accidents ☐ ☐
NOTES: ______
______</td><td>DAY/DATE: ______
Enema ☐ Laxative ☐
Overnight: Wet ☐ Dry ☐
Daytime: SP ☐ Accidents ☐ ☐
NOTES: ______
______</td></tr>
<tr><td>DAY/DATE: ______
Enema ☐ Laxative ☐
Overnight: Wet ☐ Dry ☐
Daytime: SP ☐ Accidents ☐ ☐
NOTES: ______
______</td><td>DAY/DATE: ______
Enema ☐ Laxative ☐
Overnight: Wet ☐ Dry ☐
Daytime: SP ☐ Accidents ☐ ☐
NOTES: ______
______</td><td>DAY/DATE: ______
Enema ☐ Laxative ☐
Overnight: Wet ☐ Dry ☐
Daytime: SP ☐ Accidents ☐ ☐
NOTES: ______
______</td><td>DAY/DATE: ______
Enema ☐ Laxative ☐
Overnight: Wet ☐ Dry ☐
Daytime: SP ☐ Accidents ☐ ☐
NOTES: ______
______</td><td>DAY/DATE: ______
Enema ☐ Laxative ☐
Overnight: Wet ☐ Dry ☐
Daytime: SP ☐ Accidents ☐ ☐
NOTES: ______
______</td></tr>
<tr><td>DAY/DATE: ______
Enema ☐ Laxative ☐
Overnight: Wet ☐ Dry ☐
Daytime: SP ☐ Accidents ☐ ☐
NOTES: ______
______</td><td>DAY/DATE: ______
Enema ☐ Laxative ☐
Overnight: Wet ☐ Dry ☐
Daytime: SP ☐ Accidents ☐ ☐
NOTES: ______
______</td><td>DAY/DATE: ______
Enema ☐ Laxative ☐
Overnight: Wet ☐ Dry ☐
Daytime: SP ☐ Accidents ☐ ☐
NOTES: ______
______</td><td>DAY/DATE: ______
Enema ☐ Laxative ☐
Overnight: Wet ☐ Dry ☐
Daytime: SP ☐ Accidents ☐ ☐
NOTES: ______
______</td><td>DAY/DATE: ______
Enema ☐ Laxative ☐
Overnight: Wet ☐ Dry ☐
Daytime: SP ☐ Accidents ☐ ☐
NOTES: ______
______</td></tr>
<tr><td>DAY/DATE: ______
Enema ☐ Laxative ☐
Overnight: Wet ☐ Dry ☐
Daytime: SP ☐ Accidents ☐ ☐
NOTES: ______
______</td><td>DAY/DATE: ______
Enema ☐ Laxative ☐
Overnight: Wet ☐ Dry ☐
Daytime: SP ☐ Accidents ☐ ☐
NOTES: ______
______</td><td>DAY/DATE: ______
Enema ☐ Laxative ☐
Overnight: Wet ☐ Dry ☐
Daytime: SP ☐ Accidents ☐ ☐
NOTES: ______
______</td><td>DAY/DATE: ______
Enema ☐ Laxative ☐
Overnight: Wet ☐ Dry ☐
Daytime: SP ☐ Accidents ☐ ☐
NOTES: ______
______</td><td>DAY/DATE: ______
Enema ☐ Laxative ☐
Overnight: Wet ☐ Dry ☐
Daytime: SP ☐ Accidents ☐ ☐
NOTES: ______
______</td></tr>
<tr><td>DAY/DATE: ______
Enema ☐ Laxative ☐
Overnight: Wet ☐ Dry ☐
Daytime: SP ☐ Accidents ☐ ☐
NOTES: ______
______</td><td>DAY/DATE: ______
Enema ☐ Laxative ☐
Overnight: Wet ☐ Dry ☐
Daytime: SP ☐ Accidents ☐ ☐
NOTES: ______
______</td><td>DAY/DATE: ______
Enema ☐ Laxative ☐
Overnight: Wet ☐ Dry ☐
Daytime: SP ☐ Accidents ☐ ☐
NOTES: ______
______</td><td>DAY/DATE: ______
Enema ☐ Laxative ☐
Overnight: Wet ☐ Dry ☐
Daytime: SP ☐ Accidents ☐ ☐
NOTES: ______
______</td><td>DAY/DATE: ______
Enema ☐ Laxative ☐
Overnight: Wet ☐ Dry ☐
Daytime: SP ☐ Accidents ☐ ☐
NOTES: ______
______</td></tr>
<tr><td>DAY/DATE: ______
Enema ☐ Laxative ☐
Overnight: Wet ☐ Dry ☐
Daytime: SP ☐ Accidents ☐ ☐
NOTES: ______
______</td><td>DAY/DATE: ______
Enema ☐ Laxative ☐
Overnight: Wet ☐ Dry ☐
Daytime: SP ☐ Accidents ☐ ☐
NOTES: ______
______</td><td>DAY/DATE: ______
Enema ☐ Laxative ☐
Overnight: Wet ☐ Dry ☐
Daytime: SP ☐ Accidents ☐ ☐
NOTES: ______
______</td><td>DAY/DATE: ______
Enema ☐ Laxative ☐
Overnight: Wet ☐ Dry ☐
Daytime: SP ☐ Accidents ☐ ☐
NOTES: ______
______</td><td>DAY/DATE: ______
Enema ☐ Laxative ☐
Overnight: Wet ☐ Dry ☐
Daytime: SP ☐ Accidents ☐ ☐
NOTES: ______
______</td></tr>
</table>

Multi-M.O.P. Tracker

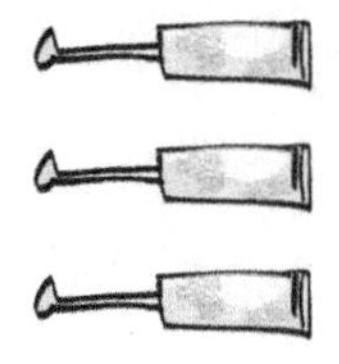

MONTHLY TOTALS:

Accident-free days ______

Accident-free nights ______

Day/Date: ______ DS Mini-Enema ☐ ☐ ☐ Overnight: Dry ☐ Wet ☐ Daytime Accidents: ☐ ☐ ☐ Notes: ______ ______ 1	Day/Date: ______ DS Mini-Enema ☐ ☐ ☐ Overnight: Dry ☐ Wet ☐ Daytime Accidents: ☐ ☐ ☐ Notes: ______ ______	Day/Date: ______ DS Mini-Enema ☐ ☐ ☐ Overnight: Dry ☐ Wet ☐ Daytime Accidents: ☐ ☐ ☐ Notes: ______ ______ 3	Day/Date: ______ DS Mini-Enema ☐ ☐ ☐ Overnight: Dry ☐ Wet ☐ Daytime Accidents: ☐ ☐ ☐ Notes: ______ ______	Day/Date: ______ DS Mini-Enema ☐ ☐ ☐ Overnight: Dry ☐ Wet ☐ Daytime Accidents: ☐ ☐ ☐ Notes: ______ ______ 5
Day/Date: ______ DS Mini-Enema ☐ ☐ ☐ Overnight: Dry ☐ Wet ☐ Daytime Accidents: ☐ ☐ ☐ Notes: ______ ______	Day/Date: ______ DS Mini-Enema ☐ ☐ ☐ Overnight: Dry ☐ Wet ☐ Daytime Accidents: ☐ ☐ ☐ Notes: ______ ______ 7	Day/Date: ______ DS Mini-Enema ☐ ☐ ☐ Overnight: Dry ☐ Wet ☐ Daytime Accidents: ☐ ☐ ☐ Notes: ______ ______	Day/Date: ______ DS Mini-Enema ☐ ☐ ☐ Overnight: Dry ☐ Wet ☐ Daytime Accidents: ☐ ☐ ☐ Notes: ______ ______ 9	Day/Date: ______ DS Mini-Enema ☐ ☐ ☐ Overnight: Dry ☐ Wet ☐ Daytime Accidents: ☐ ☐ ☐ Notes: ______ ______
Day/Date: ______ DS Mini-Enema ☐ ☐ ☐ Overnight: Dry ☐ Wet ☐ Daytime Accidents: ☐ ☐ ☐ Notes: ______ ______ 11	Day/Date: ______ DS Mini-Enema ☐ ☐ ☐ Overnight: Dry ☐ Wet ☐ Daytime Accidents: ☐ ☐ ☐ Notes: ______ ______	Day/Date: ______ DS Mini-Enema ☐ ☐ ☐ Overnight: Dry ☐ Wet ☐ Daytime Accidents: ☐ ☐ ☐ Notes: ______ ______ 13	Day/Date: ______ DS Mini-Enema ☐ ☐ ☐ Overnight: Dry ☐ Wet ☐ Daytime Accidents: ☐ ☐ ☐ Notes: ______ ______	Day/Date: ______ DS Mini-Enema ☐ ☐ ☐ Overnight: Dry ☐ Wet ☐ Daytime Accidents: ☐ ☐ ☐ Notes: ______ ______ 15
Day/Date: ______ DS Mini-Enema ☐ ☐ ☐ Overnight: Dry ☐ Wet ☐ Daytime Accidents: ☐ ☐ ☐ Notes: ______ ______	Day/Date: ______ DS Mini-Enema ☐ ☐ ☐ Overnight: Dry ☐ Wet ☐ Daytime Accidents: ☐ ☐ ☐ Notes: ______ ______ 17	Day/Date: ______ DS Mini-Enema ☐ ☐ ☐ Overnight: Dry ☐ Wet ☐ Daytime Accidents: ☐ ☐ ☐ Notes: ______ ______	Day/Date: ______ DS Mini-Enema ☐ ☐ ☐ Overnight: Dry ☐ Wet ☐ Daytime Accidents: ☐ ☐ ☐ Notes: ______ ______ 19	Day/Date: ______ DS Mini-Enema ☐ ☐ ☐ Overnight: Dry ☐ Wet ☐ Daytime Accidents: ☐ ☐ ☐ Notes: ______ ______
Day/Date: ______ DS Mini-Enema ☐ ☐ ☐ Overnight: Dry ☐ Wet ☐ Daytime Accidents: ☐ ☐ ☐ Notes: ______ ______ 21	Day/Date: ______ DS Mini-Enema ☐ ☐ ☐ Overnight: Dry ☐ Wet ☐ Daytime Accidents: ☐ ☐ ☐ Notes: ______ ______	Day/Date: ______ DS Mini-Enema ☐ ☐ ☐ Overnight: Dry ☐ Wet ☐ Daytime Accidents: ☐ ☐ ☐ Notes: ______ ______ 23	Day/Date: ______ DS Mini-Enema ☐ ☐ ☐ Overnight: Dry ☐ Wet ☐ Daytime Accidents: ☐ ☐ ☐ Notes: ______ ______	Day/Date: ______ DS Mini-Enema ☐ ☐ ☐ Overnight: Dry ☐ Wet ☐ Daytime Accidents: ☐ ☐ ☐ Notes: ______ ______ 25
Day/Date: ______ DS Mini-Enema ☐ ☐ ☐ Overnight: Dry ☐ Wet ☐ Daytime Accidents: ☐ ☐ ☐ Notes: ______ ______	Day/Date: ______ DS Mini-Enema ☐ ☐ ☐ Overnight: Dry ☐ Wet ☐ Daytime Accidents: ☐ ☐ ☐ Notes: ______ ______ 27	Day/Date: ______ DS Mini-Enema ☐ ☐ ☐ Overnight: Dry ☐ Wet ☐ Daytime Accidents: ☐ ☐ ☐ Notes: ______ ______	Day/Date: ______ DS Mini-Enema ☐ ☐ ☐ Overnight: Dry ☐ Wet ☐ Daytime Accidents: ☐ ☐ ☐ Notes: ______ ______ 29	Day/Date: ______ DS Mini-Enema ☐ ☐ ☐ Overnight: Dry ☐ Wet ☐ Daytime Accidents: ☐ ☐ ☐ Notes: ______ ______

Made in the USA
Middletown, DE
12 November 2024